KERATOPLASTIES – SURGICAL TECHNIQUES AND COMPLICATIONS

Edited by **Luigi Mosca**

Keratoplasties – Surgical Techniques and Complications
Edited by Luigi Mosca

Published by InTech

Janeza Trdine 9, 51000 Rijeka, Croatia

Publishing Process Manager Dragana Manestar

Technical Editor Teodora Smiljanic

Cover Designer InTech Design Team

Additional hard copies can be obtained from orders@intechopen.com

Keratoplasties – Surgical Techniques and Complications, Edited by Luigi Mosca
p. cm.
ISBN 978-953-307-809-0

For EU product safety concerns:
IN TECH d.o.o., Prolaz Marije Krucifikse Kozulić 3, 51000 Rijeka, Croatia,
info@intechopen.com or visit our website at intechopen.com.

Meet the editor

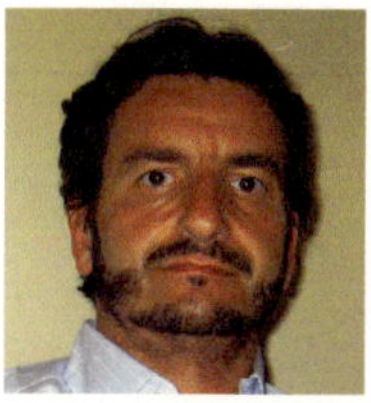

Dr Luigi Mosca (MD, PhD) graduated in Medicine at the University La Sapienza of Rome. He held a residency then research post at the Eye Clinic of the University of L'Aquila before gaining his degree in Ophthalmology and becoming a practicing Ophthalmologist – first at the Department of Ophthalmology of the A. Gemelli Polyclinic of the Catholic University of "Sacro Cuore" of Rome, then as Chief of the Cornea and Refractive Surgery Service. He is Professor of the School of Ophthalmology of Catholic University of Sacro Cuore. He is author of several scientific works in the field of Ophthalmology, refractive surgery, and corneal transplantation.

Contents

Preface

The practice of this subspecialty in ophthalmology diversifies each day, and grows with new surgical techniques and therapeutic approaches to corneal pathologies. This book on keratoplasties, divided into three sections, may perhaps seem too undemanding to some, but all the new therapeutic and surgical techniques are well approached in these chapters.

The long-lasting penetrating keratoplasty (PK) technique has shown to have good results, both anatomical and optical, leading to better visual outcomes despite other keratoplasty techniques, maintaining its place in corneal transplant surgery until today, especially in cases of infectious disease of the cornea. Moreover, for a long time, PK relegated lamellar keratoplasty (LK) techniques to primarily tectonic indications due to poor visual results. The development of new technologies (diamond knives, microkeratomes, lasers) and the creation of new surgical techniques (descemeting and predescemeting techniques) leading to better interfaces, have given a new impulse to lamellar keratoplasty surgery in the last years. Deep anterior lamellar keratoplasty (DALK) and the Descemet stripping endothelial keratoplasty (DSEK), less invasive and equally effective both in anatomical and visual outcomes, are the leading techniques for most corneal pathologies in preference to the PK today.

This edition is in an electronic format, allowing universal access to everybody regardless of the time of day or setting, portability, and speed of information access. Such features help to reduce the time needed for research, showing more feasibility for all readers.

The main purpose of this book is to show the different therapeutic and surgical techniques to treat corneal pathologies, as well as analyzing the postoperative complications of the different treatments.

I hope that this book can serve as a good tool to all students approaching the field of corneal transplantation, and to all practitioners working in the field of corneal transplantation as a contribution to improvement in care for patients with corneal disease.

Luigi Mosca, MD
Catholic University "Sacro Cuore", Rome,
Italy

Part 1

Penetrating Keratoplasty

1

Clinical Indications for Penetrating Keratoplasty and Epidemiological Study in Teaching Hospitals of Birjand Medical University from 1999 to 2006

Mohammad Hossien Davari[1] and Hoda Gheytasi[2]
[1]Vali-Asre Hospital,
Birjand University of Medical Sciences and Health Services, Birjand,
[2]Birjand University of Medical Sciences, Birjand,
Iran

1. Introduction

The cornea is normally a clear layer of tissue covering the front of the eye, similar to a watch crystal. Its purpose is to refract or bend light rays as they enter the eye, allowing them to focus on the retina (1, 2).

Corneal diseases are a significant cause of visual impairment and blindness in the developing world [3] Penetrating keratoplasty (PK) offers hope for visual rehabilitation in many such cases (3).

Corneal transplantation, also known as corneal grafting or penetrating keratoplasty, is a surgical procedure where a damaged or diseased cornea is replaced by donated corneal tissue which has been removed from a recently deceased individual having no known diseases which might affect the viability of the donated tissue (1, 4). Corneal transplantation has two major types, penetrating keratoplasty (P.K) in which the full thickness of cornea is replaced and lamellar keratoplasty (L.K) in which a portion of cornea is replaced. The term PK commonly refers to surgical replacement of a portion of the corneal with that of a donor eye. LK surgery consists of placing a partial thickness donor corneal graft in a recipient corneal bed that is prepared by lamellar dissection of diseased anterior stoma corneal tissue (5, 6).

In Worldwide, Corneal transplant is one of the most common transplant procedures although approximately 100,000 procedures are performed each year; some estimates report that 10,000,000 people are affected by various disorders that would benefit from corneal transplantation. In some situations such as scar, edema, thinning and severe distortion there is no treatment other than corneal transplantation (7, 8).

The decline of certain disorders due to changes in surgical practice, and the emergence of new surgical techniques have largely influenced the changing trend. The indications for PK have continued to change since 1940 (9-10), and investigators have studied the changing trends over the past few decades (9-13).

Indications for corneal transplantation include the following:

Optical: To improve visual acuity by replacing the opaque or distorted host tissue by clear healthy donor tissue. The most common indication in this category is pseudophakic bullous keratopathy, followed by keratoconus, corneal degeneration, keratoglobus and dystrophy, as well as scarring due to keratitis and trauma.

Tectonic/reconstructive: To preserve corneal anatomy and integrity in patients with stromal thinning and descemetoceles, or to reconstruct the anatomy of the eye, e.g. after corneal perforation.

Therapeutic: To remove inflamed corneal tissue unresponsive to treatment by antibiotics or anti-virals.

Cosmetic: To improve the appearance of patients with corneal scars that have given a whitish or opaque hue to the cornea.

To update these trends and also to provide information for the prevention of corneal blindness we report the indication causes for penetrating keratoplasty (PK) in Teaching Hospitals of Medical Birjand University from 1999 to 2006.

2. Methodology

A retrospective analysis of the records of 120 patients, who underwent PK at the Emam-reza and Vali-asr teaching hospitals of Birjand University during 7- year period from 1999 to 2006, was performed.

All surgeries were performed by one expert surgeon using the same procedure and there were no intra-operative complications. Preoperative examinations consisted of visual acuity, refractive error and slit-lamp examination. Patient's pre-operative information included age, sex, systemic disease, lid abnormalities, pre-existing ocular surface disease and corneal vascularization, surgical indications and preoperative medications. The data of the last examination including uncorrected visual acuity (UCVA), refractive error, intra-ocular Pressure (IOP), graft clarity, any episode of endothelial graft rejection during the follow-up, also, suturing technique and intraoperative complications were recorded.

graft failure and recurrence of MCD in the transplanted cornea were compiled Patients were followed up for a minimum of 2 years .This data were analyzed regarding sex, age, indication, job and location of the patient. Statistical significance was determined using X2 analysis and descriptive statistic measures including percentiles, mean and standard deviation were calculated. Personal information of patients was not disclosed and the data sheets were anonymous.

The donor lenticule was secured to the recipient corneal rim with 10-0 monofilament nylon sutures. The suturing techniques consisted of interrupted (16 separate sutures), single running (with 16 bites), and combined (8 separate sutures and a 16-bite running suture).

At the end of the operation, subconjunctival gentamicin 20 mg and betamethasone 4 mg were injected. Postoperatively, the patients were medicated with topical betamethasone 0.1% and choloramphenicol eye drops four times a day. Antibiotic eye drop was discontinued after 7 to 10 days and betamethasone eye drop was gradually tapered over 4 months.

Selective suture removal was performed for any suture-related problems and for control of astigmatism, based on topography, from four month onward. Suture removal was completed between 12 and 18 months after the date of the surgery. Patients were examined on 1st, 2nd, 3rd and 7th days and then every week up to one month, every 2 weeks up to 2 months, monthly up to 4 months, and every 2 months thereafter. Finally, Two months after complete suture removal, patients were reevaluated.

3. Result

A total of 120 patients underwent PK operations during the 7-year study period. From 120 patients; 86(71/66%) were male and 34(28/33%) were female. The mean patient's age was 53 years with a standard deviation (SD) of 20.9 and a median of 59 years. The mean age of males was 51/3±21.5 and for women was 57/2±19/1. (P=0.26)
And also, the average age of rural patients was 61± 17.4 and urban patients were 42.7 ± 20.7, in statistically, there is a significantly difference between the average age of rural patients group in compared with average age of urban patients group. (p=0.001).
The main indications cause keratoplasty were corneal locuma 75(62.5%), keratoconus 23(19.16%) and others (Bolus keratopaty + corneal dystrophy) 22(18.34%). (p=0.001) (Table1).

Job Groups	corneal locum	keratoconus	The else
1) Farmers-animal husbandman	29(76%)	---------------	9(24%)
2) Simple worker -Artisan	7(71.4%)	2(18.18%)	2 (18.18%)
3) Staff-Driver-carpet weaver	12(66.66%)	4(22.22%)	2(11.11%)
4) Housewife-Not busy	25(68%)	4(11.11%)	7(19.44%)
5) Students	2(9.1%)	13(76.47%)	2(11.76%)
Total	75(62.5%)	23(19.16%)	22(18.34%)

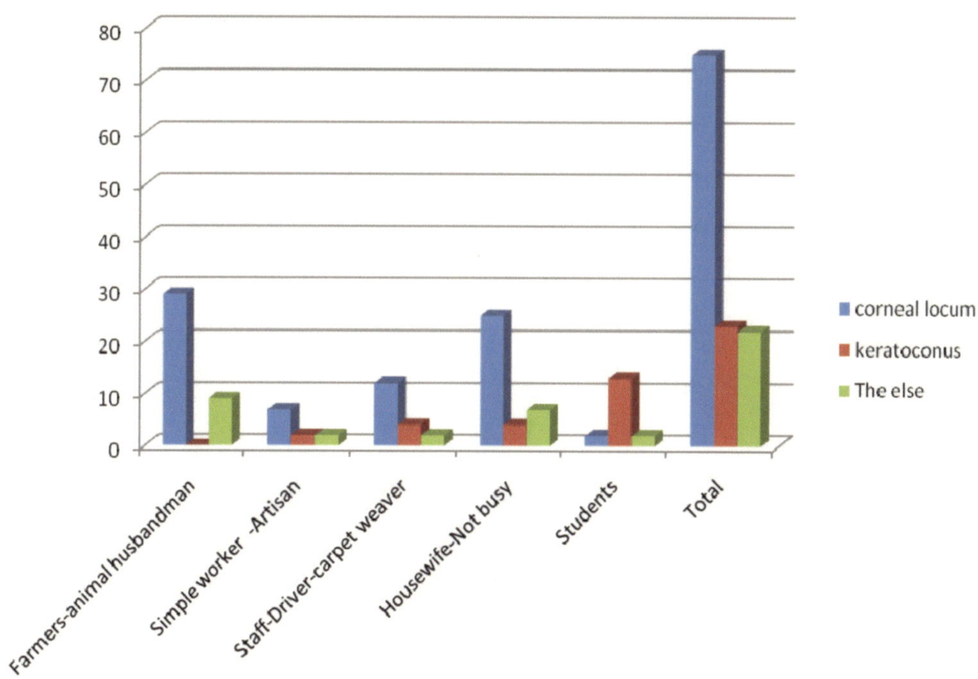

Table 1. Evaluation of indication cause of keratoplasty in Job groups

The major job for keratoplasty group was agriculture 29(76%) and housekeeping(not busy) 25(68%). because of frequent presence of corneal infectious and traumatic insults such as trachoma, herpes simplex and bacterial ulcers and trauma with Thorn barberry and ocular adnexal infection, it may be the most important cause of corneal scarring in our studies.
In corporation for indication cause of keratoplasty, there was a significantly difference between the rural patients group and urban patients groups, as shown in (table 2) (P=0.0015) but no significant sex difference was found for the cause of keratoplasty in diagnostic categories {P=0.563}.Table3
similar to this finding, studies for indication cause of keratoplasty according to age showed a significantly difference between the age and cause of PK (P=0.001) In other words, in The ages under 25 years old the main diagnoses were keratoconus (75%)15,and in The ages over 25 years old the main diagnoses were Corneal locum (Table 4).

Residence	City	village
Corneal locuma	(54.72%)29	(68.66%)46
Keratoconus	(32.07%)17	(8.95%)6
The else	(13.21%)7	(22.39%)15
Total	(100%)53	(100%)67
P=0/015 df=2 value=8/381		

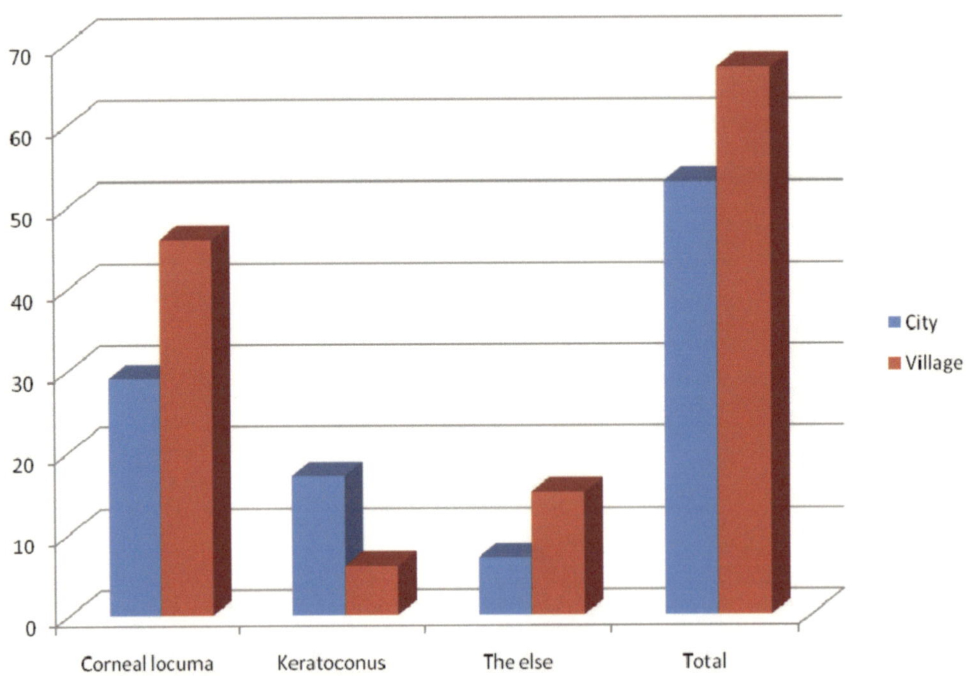

Table 2. Relationship between cause of PK and Residence

Sex	Male	Female
Corneal locuma	(61.63%)53	(64.70%)22
Keratoconus	(23.25%)20	(14.71%)5
The else	(15.12%)13	(20.59%)7
Total	(100%)86	(100%)34
P=0/563	df=2	Value:1/151

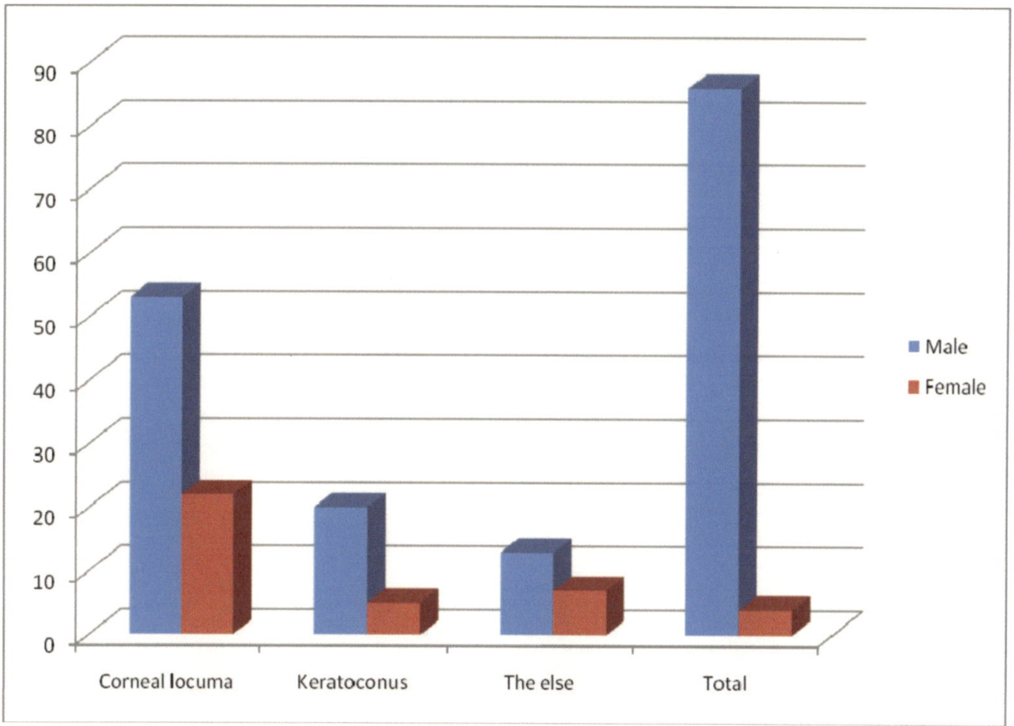

Table 3. Relationship between cause of PK and sex groups

4. Discussion

Penetrating keratoplasty can visually rehabilitate many of those who suffer from blindness or visual impairment due to corneal diseases. The prognosis of the outcome, however, is dependent on the pathology responsible for causing corneal blindness or visual impairment. [13][14][15] The purpose of our study was to document the indications for PK in Teaching Hospitals of Medical Birjand University which is a major referral centre for the treatment of corneal diseases in the Iran -Birjand .

In this study we found that the leading indications for PK were corneal scar (43%), keratoconus (20%), bullous keratopathy (16%), and corneal dystrophy and degeneration (11%). In other words, the most common indication for PK was corneal scarring and

Age groups	11-25	26-45	Up to 46
Number / Cause of pk	**19**(15.83%)	25(20.83%)	76(63.34%)
Corneal locuma	(15%)3	(54.55%)12	(76.92%)60
Keratoconus	(75%)15	(31.82%)7	(1.28%)1
The else	(7.10%)2	(13.63%)3	(21.80%)17
Total	(100%)20	(100%)22	(100%)78
P=0/001	df=4	value=40/234	

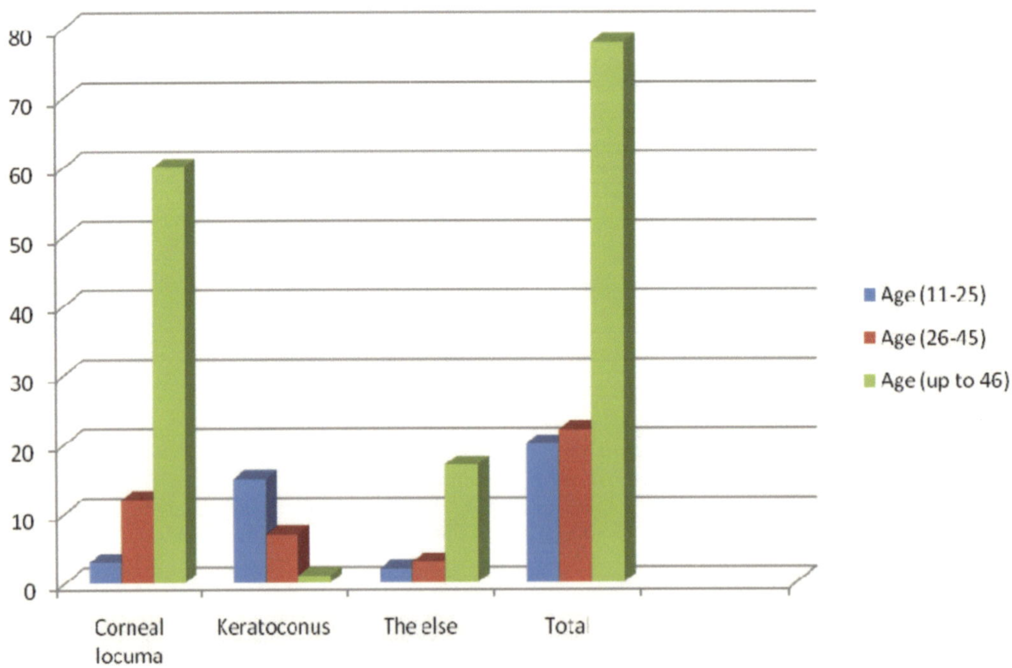

Table 4. Comparison of cause of PK in age groups

keratoconus. Similar to this finding, studies in Nakorn hospital (17)showed that The leading indications for penetrating keratoplasty, in order of decreasing frequency, were bullous keratopathy (28.9%), corneal scar (22.2%), corneal dystrophy and degeneration (20.0%), corneal ulcer (17.8%), re-graft (8.9%), and trauma (2.2%)(17). In other words, pseudophakic bullous keratopathy and corneal scar were the most common indications (17). In the study in French in 2001 pseudophakic bullous keratopathy (27.7%), keratoconus (25.3%), was the most common indication (18). In Atlanta in 2001 study showed reoperative graft (29.1%), bullous keratopathy (21.5%), keratoconus (23%), corneal scar (19%), was the most common indication (19). In the study in Iran (Teaching Hospital of Medical yazd University) between 1992 and 1996, The most common indication for PK was keratoconus (31%), corneal scar

(27%), pseudophakic bullous keratopathy and corneal dystrophies (20). The difference in our results and them can be explained by the more frequent presence of corneal infectious and traumatic insults such as trachoma, herpes simplex and bacterial ulcers. Dobbin has reported trauma as the main cause of corneal scarring but trauma with Thorn barberry and ocular adnexal infection may be more important causes of corneal scarring in our study.
Also, the decreases of bullous keratopathy disorders are due to changes in surgical practice, and the emergence of new surgical techniques.
The rate of corneal transplant rejection in most studies is between 9.9 and 17.2% but we had a failure rate of 12.3% because of poor prognosis factors in most scarred corneas such as deep vascularization and eyelid and conjunctiva defects.
There is no significant difference in the indications and outcome of corneal transplantation between males and females as could be expected (12) but other studies may show a predominance of keratoconus and trauma in males and Fuchs' dystrophy in females as indication for corneal transplantation (16).

5. Conclusions

Corneal scar and Keratoconus is the most common indication for PK in teaching hospitals of Birjand Medical University, Iran. These findings were in agreement with data reported in recent literature in Iran.

6. References

[1] Godeiro KD, Coutinho AB, Pereira PR, Fernandes BF, Cassie A, Burnier MN Jr.*Histopathological diagnosis of corneal button specimens: an epidemiological study.* Ophthalmic Epidemiol. 2007 Mar-Apr;14(2):70-5.

[2] Kanavi MR, Javadi MA, Sanagoo M. *Indications for penetrating keratoplasty in Iran. Cornea.* 2007 Jun; 26(5):561-3

[3] Thylefors B, Negrel AD, Pararajasegaram R, Dadzie KY. Global data on blindness. *Bull WHO* 1995;73:116-21

[4] Vail A, Gore SM, Bradley BA, Easty DL, Rogers CA, Armitage WJ. *Influence of donor and histocompatibility factors on corneal graft outcome. Transplantation.* 1994;58(11):1210-6.

[5] Sony P, Sharma N, Sen S, Vajpayee RB. *Indications of penetrating keratoplasty in northern India. Cornea.* 2005 Nov;24(8):989-91.

[6] Cosar CB, Sridhar MS, Cohen EJ, Held EL, Alvim PT, Rapuano CJ, et al. Indications for penetrating keratoplasty and associated procedures, 1996-2000. Cornea. 2002; 21(2):148-51.

[7] Eye Bank Association of America. 2003 Eye Banking Statistical Report. Washington, DC: Eye Bank Association of America.

[8] Human organ and tissue transplantation. Report by the Secretariat. Executive Board, EB112/5, 112th session, Provisional agenda item 4.3. World Health Organization. May 2003. Available: http://www.who.int/gb/eb wha/pdf _files /EB 112/eeb1125.pdf (accessed 2004 Oct 11).

[9] *Kervick GN, Shepherd WFI. Changing indications for penetrating keratoplasty. Ophthalmic Surg 1990; 21:227*

[10] *Haamann P, Jensen OM, Schmidt P: Changing indications for penetrating keratoplasty, Acta Ophthalmol (Copenh).* 1994 Aug;72(4):443-6.

[11] Mohamadi P, McDonnell JM, Irvine JA, McDonnell PJ, Rao N, Smith RE. *Changing indications for penetrating keratoplasty, 1984-1988.* Am J Ophthalmol. 1989;107(5):550-2.

[12] Damji KF, Rootman J, White VA, Dubord PJ, Richards JS. *Changing indications for penetrating keratoplasty in Vancouver, 1978-87.*Can J Ophthalmol.1990;25(5):243-8.

[13] Arentsen JJ, Morgan B, Green WR. Changing indications for keratoplasty. Am J Ophthalmol. 1976;81(3):313-8.

[14] Price FW, Whitson WE, Marks RG. Graft survival in four common groups of patients undergoing penetrating keratoplasty. *Ophthalmology* 1991;98:322-28

[15] Paglen FG, Fine M, Abbott RL, Webster RG. The prognosis for keratoplasty in keratoconus. *Ophthalmology* 1982;89:651-54

[16] Sugar A. An analysis of corneal endothelium and graft survival in pseudophakic bullous keratopathy. *Trans Am Ophthalmol Soc* 1989;87:762-801.

[17] Ngamti phkorns,Parasit slip: *Clinical indication for P.K in Maharaj Nakorn chaing Mai Hospital. 1996-1999;* J Med Assos 2003 Mar 86 (3) :206-211.

[18] poniard,C / Tupping / Loty B pelbose, *The French national waiting list for P.K created in 1999-patient registration dication,characterisitic and turn over,* B.J ophtalmol: 2003 Nov:26 (9) :911.

[19] Randle man JB,Song CD, Palay DA: *Indication for and out come of penetrating keratoplasty performed by resident surgeons,* America J ophtalmol.2003/ Jul/136(1):68-75.

[20] Kanavi MR, Javadi MA, Sanagoo M. Indications for penetrating keratoplasty in Iran. Cornea. 2007 Jun;26(5):561-3.

2

Therapeutic Keratoplasty for Microbial Keratitis

Ana Lilia Pérez-Balbuena, Diana Santander-García,
Virginia Vanzzini-Zago and Diego Cuevas-Cancino
*Hospital Dr. Luis Sánchez Bulnes de la Asociación Para Evitar
la Ceguera en México I.A.P.
México D.F.*

1. Introduction

Keratitis infections caused by bacteria, fungus or *Acanthamoeba* may be the most important reason for visual loss after trachoma and xerophtalmia in undeveloped and developed countries. Wilhelmus KR. 1998.

Early diagnosis and the availability of the powerful antibiotics give the opportunity of having a better control of the corneal infectious processes, mainly in those of bacteriological etiology.

However, the virulence and resistance of some bacteria Hill JC et al 1986, fungi Polack FM et al 1971 and *Acanthamoeba* Blackman HJ 1984 may progress inexorably despite the maximum therapy applied and in those cases the integrity of the ocular globe will be jeopardized and then, it will be necessary to realize a penetrating keratoplasty, by removing, totally of partially, the infectious area in the cornea in the levels where the antibiotics and defense mechanisms of the guest, might be effective.

The tectonic and therapeutic keratoplasty constitute a significant percentage of corneal transplants held in Asia and in some other under developed cities. In Singapore, it was reported a survey in which 13% of all transplants were with therapeutic or tectonic indication Tan DT, Janardhanan P 2008.

In Mexico, it was reported, in a 10 year-period, from 2001 thru 2010, out of the 3240 transplants carried out in the Hospital for the prevention of Blindness, "Asociación para Evitar la Ceguera en Mexico, IAP" Mexico City had a tectonic or therapeutic indication. If we divide the therapeutic indication from the tectonic, the percentage lows down to 2.06%

2. Indications

The therapeutic keratoplasty is a surgical procedure whose indications include the following circumstances:

a. To solve an infectious keratitis or a maximum conventional refractory inflammatory treatment.
b. To reestablish the integral structure of the ocular globe because of the risk of sclera extension, descematocele or corneal perforation (tectonic keratoplasty). In some cases, both situations occur.

The Therapeutic keratoplasty is an emergency in which the integrity of the ocular globe is at risk, contrary to the optical keratoplasty where the visual rehab is indicated after the process is already controlled.
Infectious keratitis present different clinical characteristics and history, depending on its etiology: therefore, the situations which require a penetrating keratoplasty are different from the bacterial micotic keratitis or for the *Acanthamoeba.*

2.1 Bacterial keratitis

The impact of bacterial keratitis on corneal blindness for scars, or other ocular complications is very important. In undeveloping countries for traumas risk, or in developed coutries in contact lens users, bacterial keratitis is a leading cause of corneal blindness.
Probably, the first indication for therapeutic keratoplasty, within the perforated corneal ulcers whose etiological agent is *Psedomonas aeruginosa,* especially in tropical climates, in contact lens users and in hospitalized or weak patients.
Psedomonas aeruginosa typically present as a rapidly evolving suppurative stromal infiltrate with marked mucopurulent exudate and become to corneal perforation in 24 to 48 hours because P *aeruginosa* due to colagenase production causing an important corneal stroma loss. Therapeutic keratoplasty is required too in corneal ulcers caused by others Gram negative bacteria as *Enterobacter, Serratia, klebsiella and Escherichia* that contaminate contact lens and cause a severe corneal desepitelization and ulcers with a great damage of corneal stroma with marked mucopurulent exudate frequently with similar characteristics of progressive suppurative keratitis. Fig 1,2
According to a survey published in 2007 by Ti et al, out of a revision of 92 patients (1991 to 2002) with acute infectious Keratitis in Singapore National Eye Centre, reported the *Pseudomonas aeruginosa* as the main etiological agent, responsible for the keratitis requiring therapeutic keratoplasty.

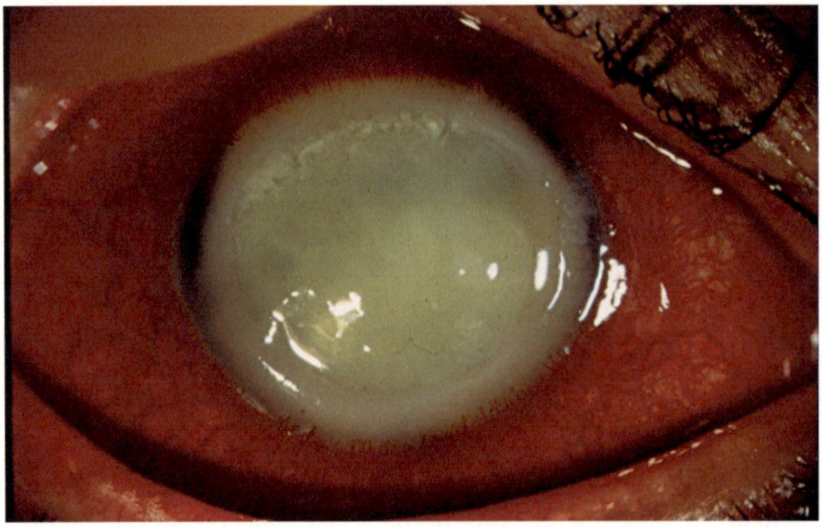

Fig. 1. Corneal ulcer caused by Gram negative, with perforation and poor response to medical treatment.

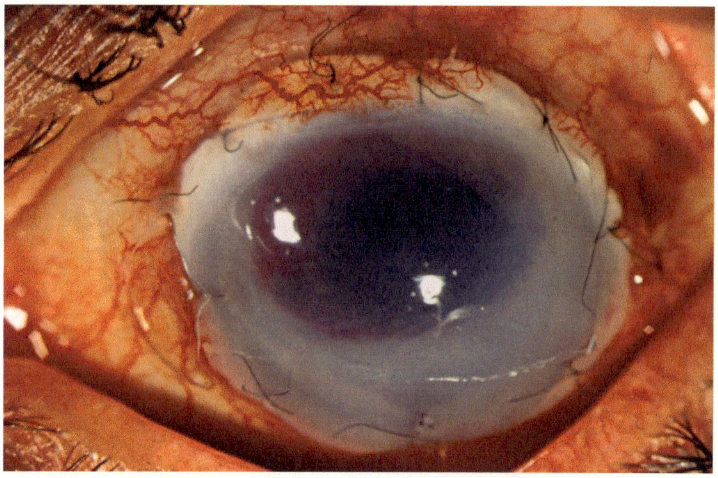

Fig. 2. The same eye 4 weecks after therapeutic sclerokeratoplasty (Courtesy of Alfredo Gomez Leal,MD Phathology Service of "Asociacion para Evitar la Ceguera en Mexico Hospital "Dr. Luis Sanchez Bulnes")

Other bacterial keratitis that might require a therapeutic keratoplasty are those infections that do not reply to a medical treatment, whose etiological agents grow slowly and behave as opportunists and sluggish and that continue to grow despite the aggressive treatment including crystalline keratopathy caused by alphahemolytic *Streptococcus* Stern GA 1993 The concomitant corneal ulcers are a sequence of severe *gonococcal* conjunctivitis Kawashima M et al 2009 and the ulcer caused atypical mycobacterium, an opportunist pathogen that produce lesions in areas where local resistance is compromised by trauma or prior surgery. Clinically, non-tuberculous *Mycobacteria* cause slow-progressing keratitis, which may mimic the indolent course of disease caused by others organism as fungi or anaerobic bacteria and frequently an delayed diagnosis progress to a severe keratitis Perez-Balbuena et al, 2010. Figs. 3, 4, 5

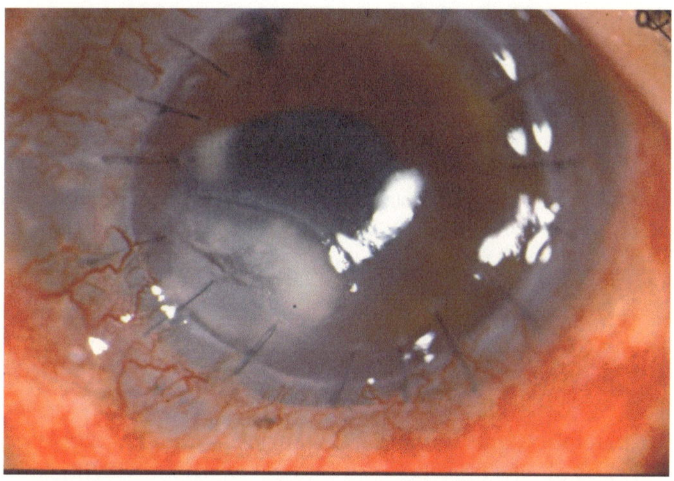

Fig. 3. *Mycobacterium chelonae* Keratitis. At initial examination, 4 weeks after penetrating keratoplasty with corneal infiltrates (3.0 X 2.0 mm) withe -gray with irregular and elevated edges in the donor-receptor interface.

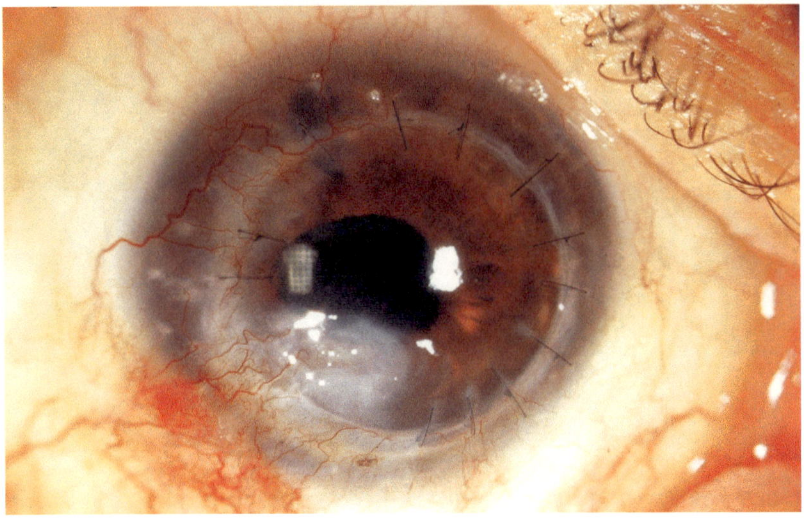

Fig. 4. Successful therapy 2 months with after topical Gatifloxacin 0.3% therapy.

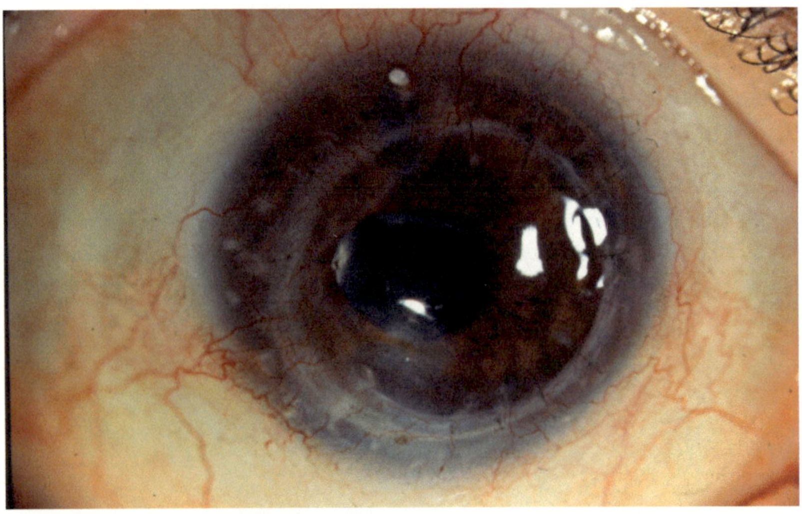

Fig. 5. Eighteen months after therapy discontinuation, corneal graft is infection-free and clear in the visual axis.

Mycobacterium keratitis is frequently present after a surgical procedure like refractive surgery (LASIK) with a slow progression to need a flap amputation or a therapeutic keratoplasty Susiyanti M, et al 2007.

Critical corneal infections occasionally requires conjunctival flap or therapeutic keratoplasty, in USA eye banking statistics identify microbial keratitis as a reason for keratoplasty in 1% of all corneal transplantation and in relation to bacterial keratitis incidence approximately 1% of USA cases of corneal infections become surgical candidates. Wilhelmus KR. 1998

In the experience obtained at the cornea service of "Dr. Luis Sánchez Bulnes" Hospital in Mexico, reported 2025 cases of infectious keratitis (survey carried out by fellow Carlos Johnson Villalobos MD. In a period from 2001 thru 2010, the causative agents were Gram positive bacteria in 67.2% cases, Gram negative bacteria in 14.91%, and fungal keratitis in 6.81% cases; In my Service, I found in 3240 keratoplasties from 2000-2010, 3.30% patients needed therapeutic keratoplasty. Figs. 6, 7

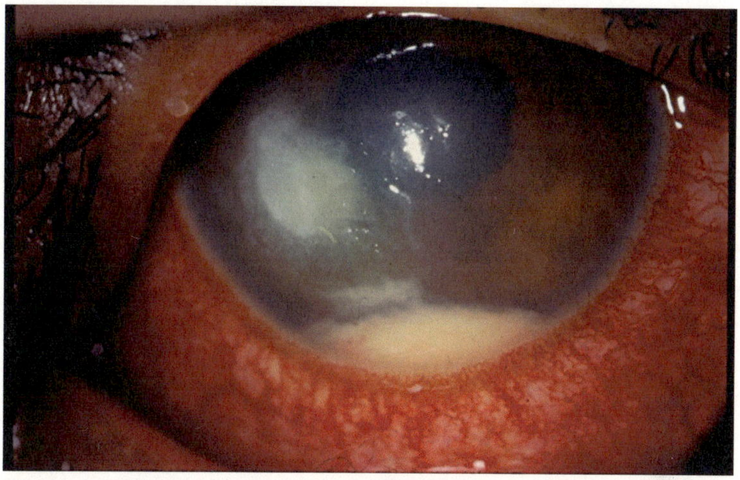

Fig. 6. Fungal keratitis (*fusarium solani*) 4 weeks evolution.

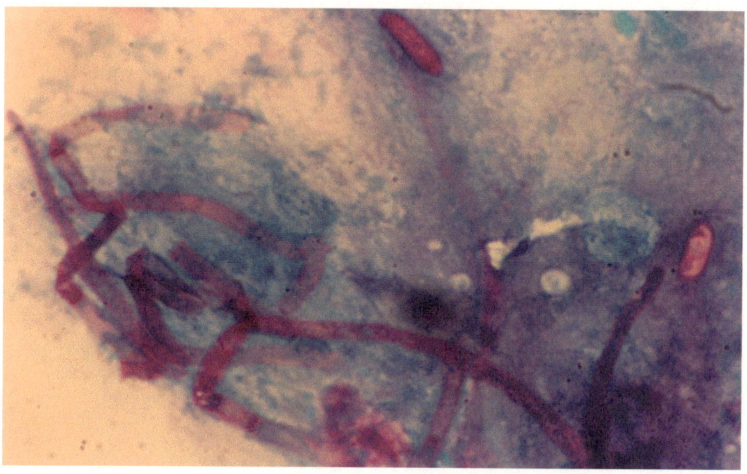

Fig. 7. Septated hyphal cells from *Fusarium solani* (Schiff stain 100X)

With the upcoming of new and more powerful antibiotics (fourth generation quinolones), the therapeutic keratoplasty is less frequently required for keratitis caused by Gram positive bacteria Al-Shehn et al. 2009, highlighted this over a 10-year period (1995-2005). They noted significant improvement in percentage of eyes achieving microbiological cure with medical therapy alone (76.0% in 1995 vs. 92.2% in 2005; p=0.002) or combining with surgical intervention (92.4% in 1995 vs. 100.0% in 2005; p=0.005).

2.2 Fungal keratitis

The therapeutic keratoplasty has an important role in the refractory mycotic ulcers treatment. In a series published by Ibrahim MM et al in 2009 in Brasil, 66 patients with

mycotic ulcer, therapeutic keratoplasty was required in 38% of cases; the most frequent isolated etiological agent was *Fusarium* in 67%, *Aspergillus* 10.5% and *Candida* 10%.
In several studies published by Perez-Balbuena et al. 2009, Vanzzini et al. **2010**, the main fungal pathogens for keratitis in Mexico are *Fusarium solani* and other species, dematiaceous fungus that include a wide group of black colony forming fungus and *Aspegillus* with several species too.

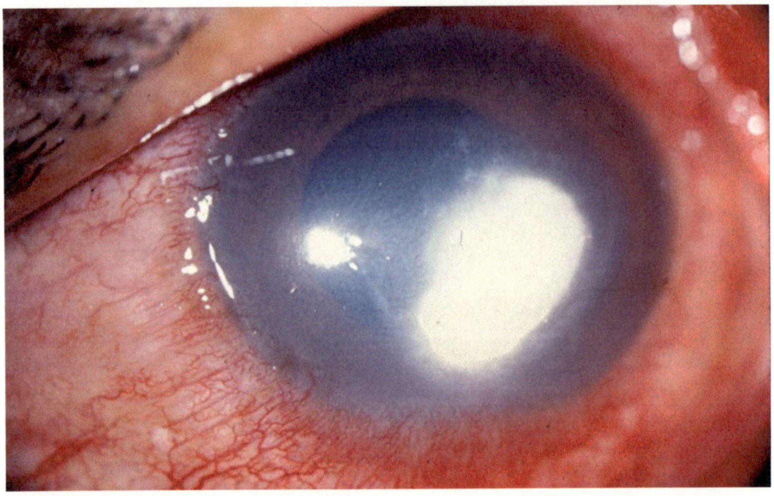

Fig. 8. *Fusarium* large corneal ulcer 10 days after injury with organic material.

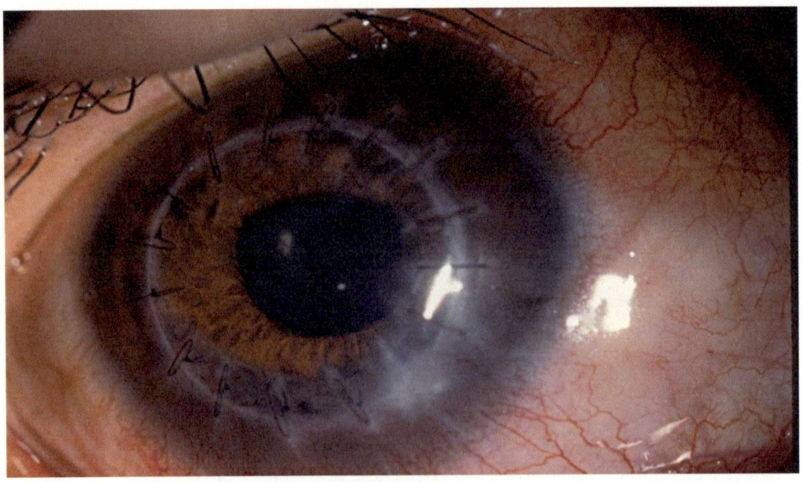

Fig. 9. Successful postoperative the same eye outcome six months after therapeutic keratoplasty loose suture after surgery

In a retrospective survey carried out from 1981 to 2001 in the Cornea Service of "Asociacion para Evitar la Ceguera en Mexico Hospital "Dr. Luis Sanchez Bulnes", we studied 120 cases of mycotic keratitis selecting 61 cases whose etiological agent was *Fusarium solani,* confirmed by the cultures. In total, 78% were male (average, age, 41.5 years) the principal risk factor was ocular trauma contaminated with organic material, dry eye, post corneal surgery in

infections and *Candida albicans* in contact lens user, and the patient came to be examined 2 to 6 weeks after the trauma.
The ulcers observed were indolent, with satellite lessons in 30% patients, irregular edges, dense infiltrate and hypopyon, ciliary injection in conjunctiva, Figs .8, 9, 10, 11 usually treated before with antibacterial drops without clinical healing.

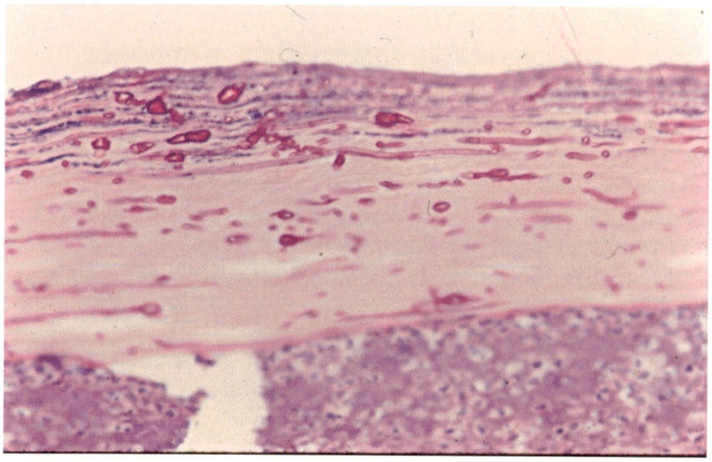

Fig. 10. Hyphal elements visible on pathologic examination of corneal button. Schiff stain (20X magnification).

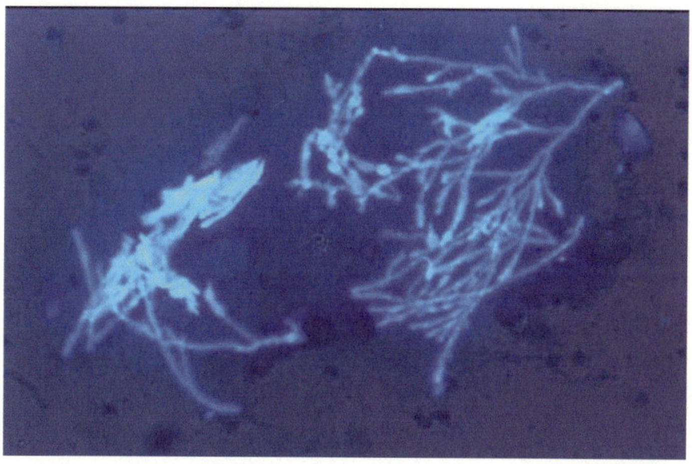

Fig. 11. Septate hyphal fungus cells in the corneal scrap smears of fungal keratitis patients, stained with calcofluor (Cellfluor) and fluorescens microscopy (20X magnification)

The antifungal treatments were started immediately after the diagnosis was confirmed in each case. The total 81% of patients were treated with monotherapy and 18.4% patients with combined antifungal therapy. As antifungal therapy, 2% ketoconazole suspensión was prepared using 200 mg tablets (Nizoral®, Janssen Cilag, Mèxico City), manually crushed to fine poder and suspended in hidroxypropylmethyl-cellulose eye drops. A total of 14 of 27 (51.2%) cases also received oral ketoconazole 200-400 mg every 24 hours. Nine patients were treated with topical itraconazole 1.0% drops (Sporanox®, Janssen-Cilag, Mèxico City) made in the same way as ketoconazole. Perez-Balbuena et al. 2009

The Fluconazole (2mg/ml Diflucan®, Pfizer) topical drops were made with intravenous solution of 2 mg/mL with <1mg/mL (0.66 mg) in final concentration using hidroxypropylmethyl-cellulose eye drops.

Severe cases were assigned to the medical and surgical treatment, using either monotherapy or combined topical antifungal treatment plus one or more surgeries. Therapeutic keratoplasty was indicated in 14/61 patients 23%. Conjuntival flap was indicated en 4 of 61 patients 6.5%, eviscearation surgeries were practiced in 14 of 61 patients 22.9%.

For medical treatment actually we use Natamycin 5% suspension in ocular droops (Miconacina® Grin laboratorios Mexico City) each 1 hour initially for two days, and after each 4 hours for 8 to 15 days upon the clinical response, we use this last dosage at least for 30 to 40 days, in cases of *Aspergillus* keratitis the medication mentioned before is associated with oral Itraconazole 100 mgs/ 12 hours. For *Candida* keratitis we use topical Voriconazole 1% (V-Fend® Pfizer Germany)) or Fluconazole 1% (Diflucan® Pfizer Germany). The indications for therapeutic keratoplasty included minimun improvement with medical therapy or high perforation risk. Table 1

	Medical / Surgical Therapy group					
Drug	n	Conjuncti-val Flap	Penetrating kerato-plasty	Tectonic kerato-plasty	Eviscera-tions	Tome of Treatment Days
Natamycin	0	0	0	0	0	0
ketoconazole	11	0	4	1	7	20.6
Miconazole	0	0	0	0	0	0
Itraconazole	3	2	2	1	2	26
Fluconazole	1	1	0	0	1	40
Ketoconazole+Natamicycin +Fluconazol	1	0	1	0	0	15
Ketoconazole+Itraconazole	1	0	1	0	0	20
Ketoconazole+Fluconazole	3	0	1	0	2	78.3
Itraconazole+ Fluconazole	2	0	2	0	0	47
Natamycin+ Fluconazole	1	1	1	0	0	170
Ketoconazole+ Miconazole	1	0	0	0	1	20
No treatment and lost follow-up	4	0	3	0	1	0
Total	28	4	15	2	14	

Table 1. Antifungal therapy used in the medical and surgery group

Killingsworth et al. 1993 obtained a 100% recovery in 15 ulcers treated with therapeutic Keratoplasty. We suggested surgical therapy with conjunctive flap or penetrating keratoplasty in advanced cases when there has been a poor response to medical therapy or a very low final visual acuity.

2.3 Acanthamoeba keratitis

The ophthalmic pathology caused by *Acanthamoeba* might produce severe and extensive corneal necrosis that tome times require therapeutic keratoplasty. The evolution of an infection becomes in a severe stromal keratitis of late diagnosis, inadequate treatment and severe consequences.

Patient with acanthamoebic keratitis are tipically young, healthy individuals, males or females are equally affected, almost all are daily contact lens wearer, or using non sterile wather for wash the contact lenses, is most frequently is an unilateral keratitis but bilateral cases have ocurred. The most important clinical sign is a severe pain even with a small epithelial dendritiform ulcer because the recurrent epithelial breakdown like an herpetic ulcer in the early stages of the infection. Some patients have a stage of disease mimicking disciform stromal keratitis and others develop radial neuritis. The occurrence of satellite lesions, stromal abscess, necrotizing inflammation, hypopyon, scleral nodules, diffuse scleritis or posterior scleral inflammation are signals of advanced infection. Figs. 12, 13 The most characteristic stromal antigen-antibody inflammatory reaction is the stromal ring formation that can consist of single, multiple or overlapping rings around the main corneal ulcer. Alizadeh H, et al 1998

The ophthalmic pathology caused by *Acanthamoeba* might produce severe and extensive corneal necrosis that tome times require therapeutic keratoplasty. The evolution of an infection becomes in a severe stromal keratitis of late diagnosis, inadequate treatment and severe consequences. Despite is rare pathology, in the last decade are incremented its frequency, associated to contact Lents user. Ficker LA et al 1993.

Before carrying out a therapeutic keratoplasty it is important to give a medical therapy and many drugs have been tested for *Acanthamoeba* infections as mentioned in the Box No 1, the most used are Chlorexidine 0.01% in aqueous solution not commercially available, Polimethylene biguanide 0.3% in aqueous solution (Brolene® UK). Oral Itraconazole 100 mgs/ 12 hours combined with topical Netilmycin 0.3% (Netira® SCIFI laboratories Italy) are actually used in our acanthamoebic keratitis patient.

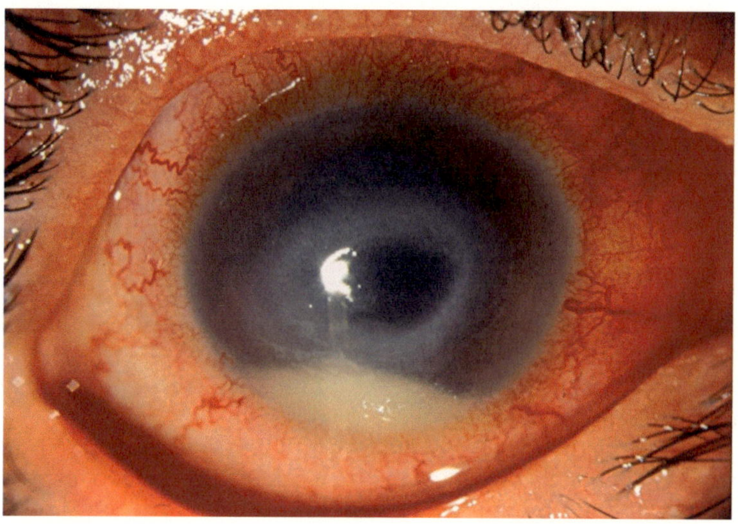

Fig. 12. *Acanthamoeba* keratitis in young and healthy female patient, 6 weeks evolution time, edema, and central ulcer.

Laboratory diagnosis are better done by visualizing cyst cells in the mucous exudate or in corneal biopsies, by stain tecniques like Giemsa Fig. 13 or Calcofluor (Cellfluor) and fluorescence ligth microscopy and by cultures C in non nutrient Pages medium with a layer of inactivated cells of *Enterobacter aerogenes.*

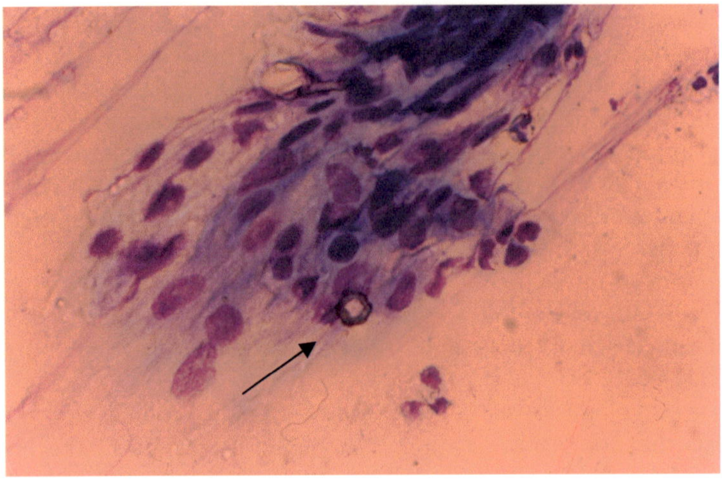

Fig. 13. *Acanthamoeba* cyst Giemsa stein, in light microscope view (20 X magnification)

Before carrying out therapeutic keratoplasty it is important to give a medical therapy and many drugs have been tested for *Acanthamoeba* infections as mentioned in the , the most used are Chlorexidine 0.01% in aqueous solution not commercially available, Polimethylene biguanide 0.3% in aqueous solution (Brolene ®UK) we used in our
Oral Itraconazole 100 mgs/ 12 hours combined with topical Netilmycin 0.3% (Netira® SCIFI laboratories Italy) are actually used in our acanthamoebic keratitis patient. Medical and surgical treatment in Keratitis by *Acanthamoeba* is controversial.
In some cases with early diagnosis these cases have been successfully treated with medical treatment without being necessary to undergo a surgical procedure of therapeutic keratoplasty. Ficker et al 1993, mention that the over life of the graft by Keratitis by *Acanthamoeba* is of poor outcome, reporting more than 50% recurrence incidence of the graft. However, in our personal opinion, the Keratoplasty continues to have a central role in the management of patients who progress or do not respond to medical treatment. The acute management of these active cases is to sterilize the infection as rapidly as posible and to dalay surgical management until the patient receives adequate antiamebic therapy.

3. Pre-surgical evaluation

When the decision has been taken to perform a therapeutic Keratoplasty, a good examination is necessary to value the following points.
To evaluate the size, depth and place of the infiltrate or corneal ulcer, if the limbos is compromised, or if there is imminent or actual perforation.
To evaluate the posterior pole under dilation, if it is possible, specially the vitreo retinal area, and when it is not possible we must realize a B Scan ultrasound and if the integrity of the ocular globe is affected by an imminent perforation it is necessary to make a Trans palpebral ecography to evaluate a probable endophtalmitis. Increased risk for endophthalmitis at the time of therapeutic keratoplasty includes the presence of fungal disease, corneal perforation and patients who have undergone previous cataract extraction.
To evaluate the presence of cataract and to carefully decide the extraction of the crystalline since this is a barrier to avoid the extension of the infectious process toward the posterior pole. It is recommended to try to keep the posterior capsule to diminish the risk of Endophthalmitis. SpeakerMG et al 1991.

Before surgery, intraocular pressure should be evaluated in eyes without a perforation. Adequate pressure control remains essential. In patients with markedly elevated intraocular pressure or in patients with a corneal perforation in which the lens-iris-diaphragm has moved forward, we give intravenous manitol to control intraocular pressure and to reduce the vitreous volume.
In eyes with a crystalline lens or posterior chamber intraocular lens, and patients with iris incarcerated in a wound, we give Pilocarpina 2% 1 hour prior to surgery, to protect the lens, and maintain a posterior lens-iris diaphragm.
We do not recommend carrying out the surgery with local anesthesia, it is much better to perform it under general anesthesia and in all cases we must maintain the arterial pressure under control to reduce the risk of expulsive choroidal hemorrhage, especially in those patients with perforation.

4. Preoperative treatment

Before therapeutic keratoplasty for infectious keratitis, the patient should be treated with topical and systemic therapy directed towards the offending microbe. This treatment applies to bacterial, fungal and *Acanthamoeba.*
Regardless of the infectious etiologies, we always recommend topical antbiotic therapy to prevent bacterial super infection.
The preoperative antibiotic prophylaxis should be broad spectrum and nontoxic to help promote reepithelization and prefer an antibiotic that penetrates into the cornea, aqueous achieve levels above to MIC_{90} of most pathogenic bacteria.
We currently use a topical fourth -generation fluoroquinolone Gatifloxacin 0.3% (Zymar^R; Allergan Inc, Irvine, CA) with a saturating dosage of one drop every 15 minutes for 1 hour before keratoplasty.

5. Donor material

Criteria for the selection of donor corneas are stringent, except in cases of large perforation when access to tissue of optimal quality is not possible. Corneal tissue of excellent grade offers the following advantages:
5.1. Healthy tissue with intact epithelium minimizes the risk of re infection in the graft and use of healthy endothelium is critical for the survival of the graft.
5.2. Compact and clear tissue helps in monitoring anterior chamber reaction during the immediate postoperative period.
Yao et al. 2003. If fresh donor tissue is not available, the use of cryopreserved tissue and donor corneas preserved in pure glycerin or water-free calcium chloride are effective substitutes in therapeutic keratoplasty to control severe fungal corneal infection and preserve the global integrity.

6. Surgical techniques

Although corneal transplantation for infections keratitis follows the basic surgical technique of penetrating keratoplasty, special attention must be given to certain details:

6.1 Preoperative procedures

We recommend general anesthesia .It is important to have a soft eye preoperatively so that problems related to positive vitreous pressure can be prevented.

Intravenous Manitol produces deturgescence of the vitreous and helps to minimize these problems.
At the time of therapeutic keratoplasty by placing the appropriate trephine over the cornea and creating an indentation in the epithelium.

6.2 Exposure

In general, we commonly use lid speculum and suture a Fleringa ring in place to provide scleral support, in cases of large ulcers that reach up to the limbus, peritomy is required and homeostasis is achieved by the use of wet-field cautery.

6.3 Host preparation bed

The goal of surgery is to excise all necrotic or infected tissue during trephination. It possible, a 1 mm rim of healthy corneal tissue should also be removed to leave a stable, no infected recipient bed.
Conjuntival peritomies should be done in cases requiring large or eccentric grafts.
The trephination of the recipient bed can be technically difficult. Careful partial-thickness trephination with a Sharp trephine is done in the absence of any perforation; in eyes with a perforation, support is obtained with cyanocrylate and viscoelastic protection and anterior chamber can be reformed and the host trephination can be performed under a more controlled environment, care should be taken to avoid exerting excessive pressure on the globe to prevent extrusion of the ocular contents a freehand dissection of the host bed may be done.

6.4 Clearing the anterior chamber of exudates

Irrigation of the anterior chamber is done using a balanced salt solution. Elimination of all exudative material from the anterior chamber helps to prevent the recurrence of infection and reduces complications such as glaucoma.
The membranes over iris are dissected gently by the irrigating cannula and are removed with forceps. Any membrane covering the iris surface should be removed very gently, and every effort should be made to arrest bleeding from the iris surface.
Intracameral antibiotics or antifungals can be used whenever they are required.
Two large peripheral iridectomies are recommended .Removal of cataracts should be deferred because the lens forms an effective barrier that prevents the spread of infection into the vitreous. When vitreous involvement is diagnosed, open sky vitrectomy is indicated. The anterior chamber is reformed with a viscoelastic substance, and the margin of the recipient bed is trimmed.

6.5 Preparation of the donor botton

The donor button should be trephined after the size of the recipient opening is measured and preparation of the host bed, because necrotic tissue may require additional trimming which may alter the size of the graft.
The donor button is punched from the endothelial side and usually 0.5-1.0 mm larger than the selected host trephine.

6.6 Suturing

The donor-recipient junction was sewn by 10-0 monofilament Nylon interrupted sutures passing though at least 70% depth of the host cornea is the preferred technique. Full thickness bites are not taken as they may form a conduit for passage of infection from the cornea into the anterior chamber. It is not uncommon to use greater number of sutures than conventional technique of keratoplasty (16 Sutures).Table 2

Age	50,90 ± 16,298 years old
Sex	68,7 % (♂)
Type penetrating keratoplasty	98.5% QPP vs.1.5% Lamelar
Endophthalmitis	11,9 %
Perforation	50,7 %
Survival graft	10,08 ± 15,97 months
Size of the donor	8,80 ± 0,19 mm.
Size receiver	8,17 ± 0,13 mm.

Table 2. Profile of infectious keratitis 2025 cases, during 10 years (2000-2010) in 14.65% cases with therapeutic keratoplasty in advanced process, dates of "Asociación Para Evitar la Ceguera en México Hospital "Dr. Luis Sanchez Bulnes"

7. Postoperative management

Immediate postoperative treatment focuses on prevention of recurrence of infection and hastening the complete epithelization of the graft.

Bacterial keratitis.

Systemic antimicrobial: Initiate 1 day prior, continue for 2 weeks.
Topical antibiotic: With most sensitivity, given hourly and topically. Combination therapy or a broad - spectrum antibiotic for which sensitivity is unknown.
Topical corticosteroids: Every 1 or 2 hours initially. Given judiciously.
Cycloplegics: Recommended to ciliary spasm and prevent synechiae.
Antiglaucoma medication: If intraocular pressure is elevated (avoid pilocarpine, prostaglandin analogues).
Tears substitutes: Frequent instillation is recommended to hasten re-epithelization.

Fungal Keratitis.

Topical antifungals: Every hour initially continue for 8-12 -weeks.
Systemic antifungals. Oral Itraconazole 200 mg two times daily continues for 2 -6weeks.
Corticosteroids: Only under extremely special conditions. Given judiciously.
Cyclosporine: Topical drops 0.5%
Cycloplegics: Recommended to ciliary spasm and prevent synechiae.
Antiglaucoma medication: If intraocular pressure is elevated (avoid pilocarpine, prostaglandin analogues).
Tears substitutes: Frequent instillation is recommended to hasten re-epithelization.

***Acanthamoeba* keratitis.**

Topical amoebicidal: Drugs - every 1 to 2 hours.
Systemic antifungal: Oral Itraconazole 200 mg two times daily.
Topical Corticosteroids: Given judiciously.
Cycloplegics. Recommended to ciliary spasm and prevent synechiae.
Antiglaucoma medication: If intraocular pressure is elevated (avoid pilocarpine, prostaglandin analogues).
Tears substitutes frequent instillation is recommended to hasten re-epithelization

Box 1. Guidelines for postoperative management of terapeutic keratoplasty

Appropriate antimicrobial therapy must be continued postoperatively until the corneal epithelium has healed

The general guidelines for postoperative management are shown in (Box 1). Therapy may be guided by histopathological and microbiological evaluation of the excised corneal tissue.

8. Complication

Postoperative complications after therapuetic keratoplasty are virtually the same as in other situations, except the prevalence is greater.

Depending on the time of onset, complications can be divided in early- onset complications (within 2 weeks) and late-onset complications. The early postoperative period may be complicated with wound leak, shallow anterior chamber, hyphema, anterior uveitis, elevated intraocular pressure, persistent epithelial defect and re- infection of the graft. Late postoperative complications include cataract, glaucoma, graft failure secondary to rejection, infection or endothelial decompensation and phthisis bulbi. Table 3

COMPLICATION	%
Corneal Decompesation/ primary failure	37.31
Recidive	31.34
Persistent epithelial defect	23.88
Glaucoma	22.38
Refractory to treatment reyect	7.46
Cataract	7.46
Ptisis bulbi	2.98
Corneal melting	4.47
Seidel	1.49
Retinal detachment or DC	1.49
Cellulitis orbitaria	1.49
Primary failure	26.66
Corneal decompensation Flat anterior chamber	10.44 1.70

Table 3. Therapeutic keratoplasty Complications of infectious keratitis 2025 cases, during 10 years (2000-2010) in 14.65% cases with therapeutic keratoplasty in advanced process, dates of "Asociación Para Evitar la Ceguera en México Hospital "Dr. Luis Sanchez Bulnes", some patient had one or two complications.

8.1 Early-onset complications

8.1.1 Seidel

This is an avoidable complication if the surgical technique is careful and the wound is well constructed The best way to prevent wound leaks is to ensure meticulous wound apposition at the end of the procedure. Promptly resuturing is recommended if non surgical attempts like patching or contact lens bandage fail to seal the leak. Prolonged contact between the donor cornea and the iris, lens, or IOL may result in irreversible complications and sequel. In our experience resuture was needed in 1, 49% of therapeutic keratoplasty.

8.1.2 Shallow or flat anterior chamber

This is a generally avoidable complication with a watertight wound. At the end of the surgery is critical that we ensure the integrity of the wound. Shallow or flat anterior chamber if present, should be managed as soon as possible to avoid synechiae formation which may result in irreversible endothelial cell loss and consequently early graft failure. In our center we needed to reform the anterior chamber either with BSS or with viscoelastic substances in 1, 7 % of the cases.

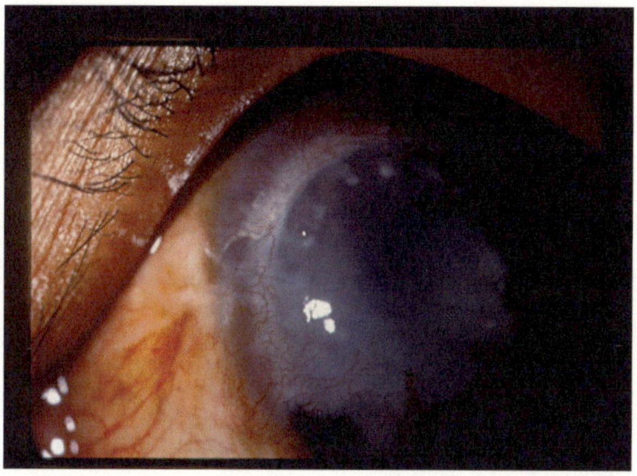

Fig. 14. Flat anterior chamber in this patient with synechiae formation post therapeutic keratoplasty

8.1.3 Hyphema

Surgical trauma on an eye with vessels on the surface of the iris or in the cornea can cause hyphema. Every effort should be done to prevent bleeding from the iris surface. Slight bleeding usually stops spontaneously with closure of the eye and return of adequate IOP. If the hemorrhage persists in the presence of an adequate IOP, then it may need to be

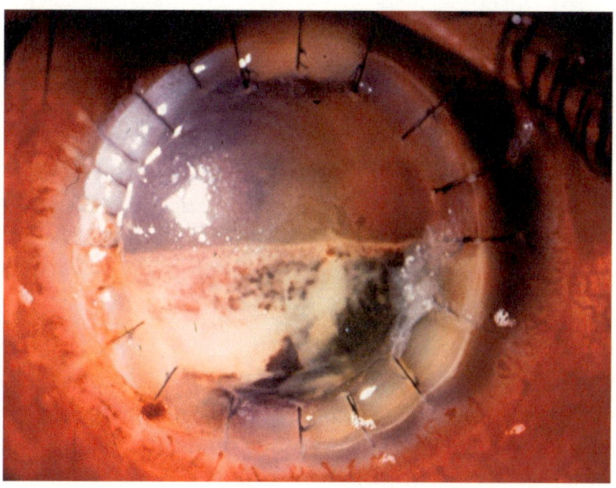

Fig. 15. Fibrine and hyphema 48 hours post keratoplasty in severe fungal ulcer (*Aspergillus flavus)*

Controlled using cautery, compression with viscoelastic, or tamponade with sponges soaked with epinephrine 1:1000. If hyphema is persistent and provokes a rise in intraocular pressure, it should be immediately evacuated. Fig. 15

8.1.4 Anterior uveitis

Infectious keratitis itself explains the great inflammation that is seen after PK in these patients. The risk of severe postoperative inflammation can be diminished by gentle manipulation during surgery and the meticulous removal of all inflammatory material of the anterior chamber. The aggressive control of postoperative inflammation is also essential for the prevention of synechiae formation. Usually the uveitis is solved with the aid of cicloplegic and corticosteroid drugs, but the latter should be used with caution in fungal and *Acanthamoeba* keratitis.

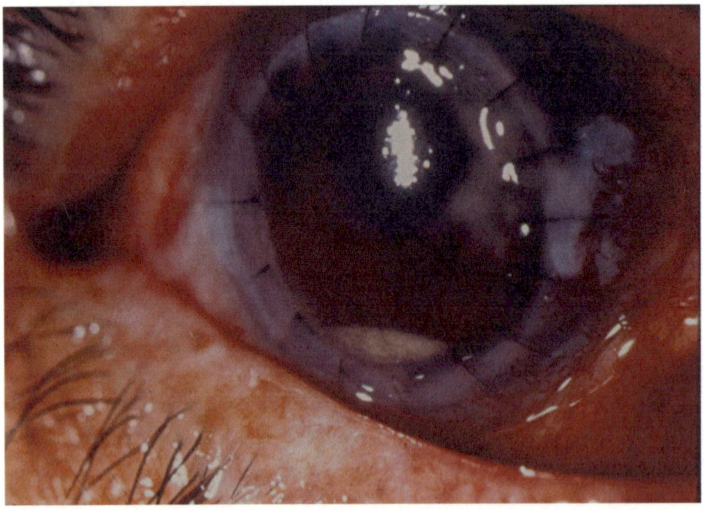

Fig. 16. Corneal ulcer by *Aspergillus flavus* ,three days Post- keratoplasty

8.1.5 Ocular hypertension

Severe inflammation causes trabeculitis and this causes elevation of the intraocular pressure. Besides peripheral anterior synechiae if present and not broken during surgery can impeed aqueous outflow and cause secondary glaucoma. Usually elevation of intraocular pressure can be controlled with beta blockers and systemic acetazolamide while the inflammation diminishes.

8.1.6 Persistent epithelial defect

Careful handling of the donor cornea intraoperatively is imperative to avoid damaging the epithelium. Good wound apposition and prevention of an overriding edge leads to better tear-film distribution and a reduced incidence of epithelial defects. A persistent epithelial defect has the potential to secondary infection thus reepithelialization and the maintenance of an intact epithelium is critical for postoperative wound healing, graft survival, and protection against infection and melting. Initial treatment requires application of topical lubricants and if it persists a permanent or temporary tarsorrhaphy early in the

postoperative period can be performed. Alternatively, botulinum A toxin injected into the elevator muscle to induce a complete ptosis, may help reduce the severity and persistence of an epithelial defect.
The use of preservative-free medication is recommended to reduce the risk of epithelial toxicity and corticosteroids may need to be decreased.

8.1.7 Recurrence

The indiscriminate use of corticosteroids postoperatively can cause recurrence of the infection, especially in micotic keratitis. In our experience we report recurrence in 31, 4%, being the most frequent cause fungal keratitis, as Rao et al 1999 reported. 50% of these recurrences needed a new PK to be free of infection. Time of recurrence varied between 1-42 days.

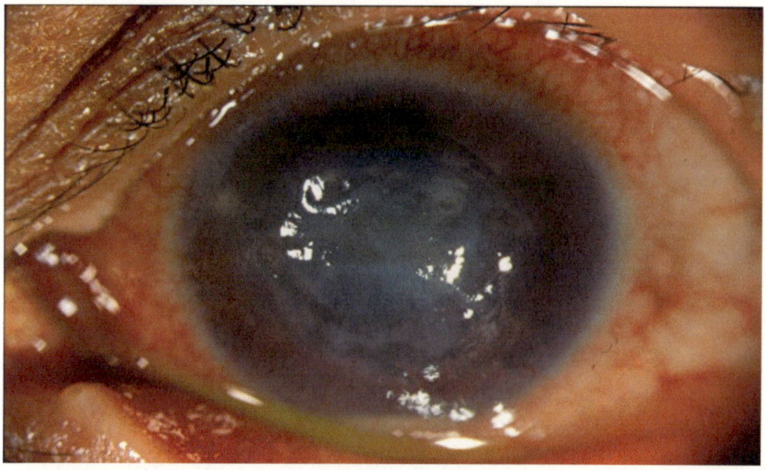

Fig. 17. Therapeutic keratoplasty, *Mycobacterium chelonae* corneal ulceration 30 Days post LASIK

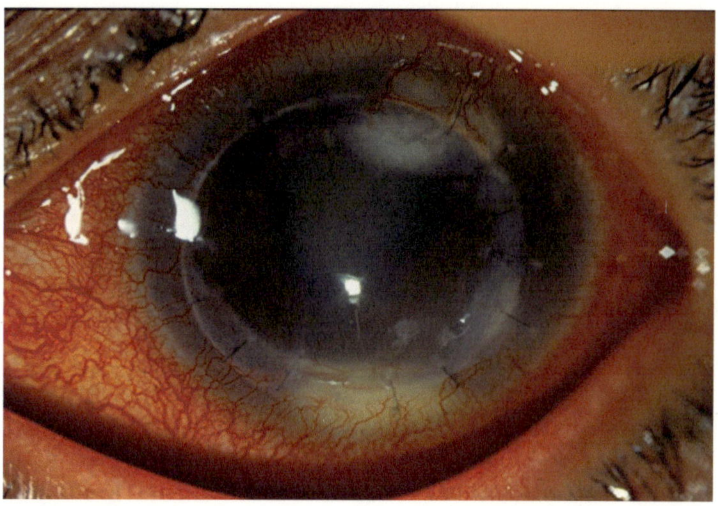

Fig. 18. Same eye showing recurrence of infection (*Mycobacterium chelonae*) Involving the entire graft

Recurrences can be avoided by performing a careful excision of the recipient cornea including all the infected material and with as adequate postoperative antibiotic and corticosteroid management. In our experience in fungal keratitis an Non tuberculous *Mycobacterium* we observed 31.34% recurrences. Fig. 17,18.

8.2 Late-onset complications

8.2.1 Secondary glaucoma

Adequate control of postoperative inflammation and careful liberation of synechiae during surgery lowers the incidence of secondary glaucoma which can endangers keratoplasty success. We found a incidence of secondary glaucoma of 22,4%. Only 4, 47% patients needed a filtering surgery to control intraocular pressure. Fig. 19.

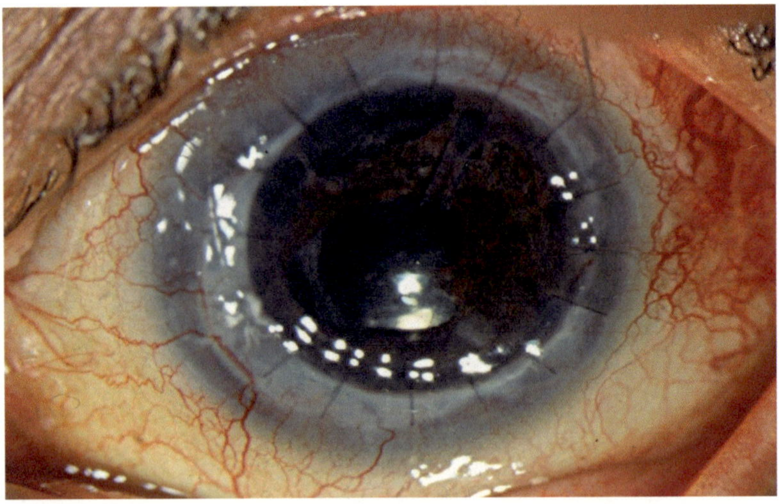

Fig. 19. Some patient needed Ahmed valvule for hypertension control

8.2.2 Cataract

As lens metabolism is dependent on the health of the eye, any ocular disease that affects the supply of oxygen and nutrients, or produces toxic substances will give rise to cataract. Also the incidence of cataract formation is higher because of the intense postoperative steroid treatment. We did find an incidence of 7, 46%.

8.2.3 Graft failure

Graft failure can be secondary to unresponding to treatment graft reject, endothelial descompensation or infection recurrence. It is much more common in therapeutic keratoplasties than in other indications. We report an incidence of 38,8%. In our center is much higher than in other reports because the quality of donor tissue in this type of keratoplasty is not as good as in optical procedures because of the relative paucity of corneal tissue in our country as well as the emergency under which this surgery is performed. Sharma et al. 2010 After the integrity of the globe is preserved and ocular inflammation has subsided, a smaller-diameter optical keratoplasty may be performed electively for visual rehabilitation

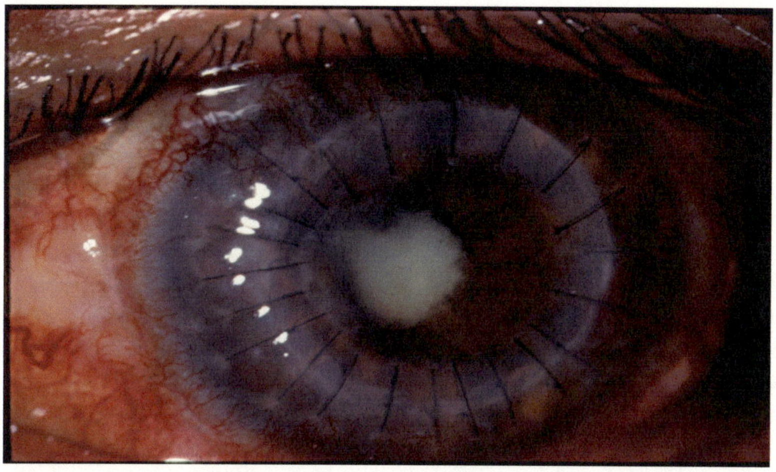

Fig. 20. Post Therapeutic keratoplasty in Candida keratitis, with clear button and cataract.

8.2.4 Phthisis bulbi

Severe inflammation causes if left untreated, can cause great alteration and disorganization of intraocular structures and atrophia. Despite all efforts to maintain globe integrity we still can find phthisis in 2, 98% of the therapeutic keratoplasties.

9. Conclusion

Therapeutic keratoplasty is generally an emergency, high-risk procedure that challenges the surgical and medical skills of the corneal surgeon. It requires meticulous attention to detail and careful postoperative monitoring. Therapeutic keratoplasty play a definitive role in the treatment of microbial keratitis refractory to medical therapy. Advances in microsurgical technique, antimicrobial therapy new and more powerful antibiotics (fourth generation quinolones), and control of inflammation have resulted in an improved prognosis for therapeutic keratoplasty in cure and improved visual outcomes.

10. References

Alizadeh H, Niderkorn Y, & McCulley J. 1998. Acanthamoebic keratitis In: *Ocular infections and Immunity*. Pepose JS,

Holland GN, Wilhelmus KR. 1062-1071. Mosby Co. 0-8016-6757-7 St Louis Missouri USA.

Al-Shehri A, Jastaneiah S, &Wagoner MD. 2009. Changing trends in the clinical course and outcome of bacterial keratitis at King Khaled Eye Specialist Hospital. *Int Ophthalmol*. 29; 143-152. ISSN 0165-5701

Blackman HJ, Rao NA, Lemp MA, & Visvesvara GS. 1984 Acanthamoeba keratitis successfully treated with penetrating keratoplasty. *Cornea*, 3:125-130. ISSN 0277-3740

Donnenfeld ED, & Solomon R. 2005 Chapter 139 Therapeutic keratoplasty, In Cornea, Krachmer, Mannis, & Holland 1695-1704. Elsevier Mosby ISBN 0323032150 Philadelphia.

Ficker LA, Kirkness C, &Wright P. 1993. Prognosis for keratoplasty in Acanthamoeba keratis. *Ophthalmology*; 100:105- 10. ISSN0161-6420

Gullapalli N, &RAO, 1999 Chapter 65 Penetrating Keratoplasty in Infectious Keratitis, IN Corneal Surgery Theory, Technique, Tissue, Frederik S, Brightbill,MD. 518-525. Mosby, ISBN 0-8151-1229-7 St Louis Missouri.

Hill JC. 1986. Use of penetrating keratoplasty in acute bacterial keratitis. *BrJ Ophthalmol,* 70: 502. ISSN 0007-1161

Ibrahim MM, Vanini R, Ibrahim FM, Ibrahim MM, Fioriti LS, Furlan EM, Provinzano LM, De Castro RS, Sousa & Rocha EM. 2009. Epidemiologic aspects and clinical outcome of fungal keratitis in southeastem Brasil. *Eur J Ophthalmol.* 19: 355-361. ISSN 1120-6721

Kawashima M, Kawakita T, & Den S. 2009. Surgical management of corneal perforation secondary to gonococcal keratoconjuntivitis. *Eye.* 23: 339-344. ISSN 0950-222X

Killingsworth DW, Stern GA, Driebe WT, Knapp, A. & Dragon DM. 1993 Results of therapeutic penetrating keratoplasty. *Ophthalmology.*100:534-541. ISSN 0161-6420

Pérez-Balbuena AL, Vanzzini-Rosano V, Valadez-Virgen Jde J. & Campos M J. 2009. Fusarium keratitis in Mexico. *Cornea.* 28 (6):626-630 July ISSN 0277-3740

Perez-Balbuena AL, Vanzzini-Zago V, Garza M, &Cuevas-Cancino D, 2010 Atypical Mycobacterium keratitis associated with penetrating keratoplasty: Case reporte of successful therapy with topical Gatifloxacin 0.3%. *Cornea,* 29(4) April. ISSN 0277-3740

Polack FM, Kaufman HF, & Newmark G. 1971.Keratomycosis medical and surgical management, *Arch Ophthalmol* 85:410. ISSN 0003-9950.

Sharma N, Vajpayee RB, Pushker N,& Vajpayee M. 2000. Infectious Cristalline kerayopathy, *CLAOJ* 26; 40-43 ISSN 1542- 2321

Sharma N, Sachdev R, Jhanji V, Titiyal JS & Vajpayee RB,2010 Therapeutic keratoplasty for microbial . Current Opinion in ophthalmology 21:293-300. ISSN 1040-8738.

Speaker MG, Menikoff JA. Prophylaxis of endophthalmitis with topical povidone iodine. Ophthalmology 98:1769- 75,1991. ISSN 0161-6420

Stern GA. infectious crystalline keratopathy (1993). *Int Ophthalmol Clin* 33 (1): 1-7. ISSN 0020-8167 Susiyanti M, Metha JS,& Tan DT. 2007. Bilateral deep anterior lamellar keratoplasty for the management of bilateral post LASIK mycobacterial keratitis. *J Cataract Refract Surg;* 33:1641-1643. ISSN0886-3350

Tan DT, Janardhanan P, Zhou H. Chan YH, Htoon HM,& Ang LP,(2008) Penetrating keratoplasty in Asian eyes: The Singapore Corneal transplant Study. *Ophthalmology.* 115:975-82 ISSN 0161-6420

Ti SE, Scott JA, Janardhanan P, &Tan DT. (2007) Therapeutic keratoplasty for advanced suppurative keratitis . *Am J Opthalmol;* 143:755-762. ISSN 0002-9394

Vanzzini Z V, Manzano-Gayosso P, Hernández-Hernández F, Méndez-Tovar L J, Gómez-Leal A, López Martínez R, (2010). Mycotic keratitis in an eye care hospital in Mexico City. *Rev. Iberoamericana Micología.* 27(2) January. 57- 61. ISSN 1130-1406

Wilhelmus KR. (1998) Bacterial keratitis, In: *Ocular infections and Immunity.*Pepose JS, Holland GN, Wilhelmus KR. 970- 1031. Mosby Co. ISSN0-8016-6757-7St Louis Missouri USA.

Yao YF, Zhang YM, Zhou P, Zhang B,Qiu W-Y, Tseng SCG 2003.Therapeutic penetrating kerathoplasty in severe fungal keratitis using cryopreserved donor corneas *Br.J Ophthalmol.*87:543-547. ISSN 0007-1161

3

Keratoplasty in Contact Lens Related Acanthamoeba Keratitis

Beata Kettesy, Laszlo Modis Jr.,
Andras Berta and Adam Kemeny-Beke
Department of Ophthalmology, Medical and Health Science Center
University of Debrecen
Hungary

1. Introduction

Acanthamoeba keratitis (AK) infection is a rather frequently occurring disease all over the world which can still cause serious or even total loss of vision despite improved diagnostic and therapeutic options. It may cause mostly keratitis, scleritis or chorioretinitis in people with competent immune systems.

It mainly affects contact lens wearers with poor hygiene. Corneal trauma due to foreign body injury and exposure to contaminated water may also be associated with *Acanthamoeba* infection.

Those with Acanthamoeba keratitis generally are immunocompetent. Nevertheless, these individuals do not develop protective immunity, and thus reinfection can occur. In the mid 1980s, an epidemic of Acanthamoeba keratitis occurred in the US which was attributed to increased contact lens use and poor lens hygiene.

Conditions promoting the disease include not only poor contact lens hygiene but also the use of home-made saline solutions and corneal abrasions (Stehr-Green at al., 1989).

In the United Kingdom, there was a marked rise in the number of cases in the first half of the 1990s, associated with the introduction and increasing popularity of disposable soft contact lenses shown to be due to irregular and/or chlorine based disinfection. After 1995 there was a decrease, perhaps resulting from an improvement in CL hygiene following the widespread dissemination of the results of a paper on Acanthamoeba keratitis as well as the gaining penetrance of new CL hygiene systems (Radford et al., 1995, 1998, 2002).

1.1 Features of Acanthamoeba

Free-living amoebae belonging to the genus *Acanthamoeba* are the causative agents of granulomatosus amoebic encephalitis, a fatal disease of the central nervous system, cutaneous lesions and sinusitis in immonodeficient patients and amoebic keratitis, a painful sight-threatening disease of the eyes in otherwise healthy individuals.

Acanthamoeba was first described by Castellani when he reported the presence of an amoeba in *Cryptococcus pararoseus* cultures. The genus *Acanthamoeba* was established later by Volkonsky in 1931 (Marciano-Cabral & Cabral, 2003).

The first suggestion that *Acanthamoeba* could cause disease in humans came in 1958 during polio vaccine safety trials. Plaques appeared in cell cultures used to prepare vaccine and were thought to be virus induced because mice and monkeys died from encephalitis following inoculation of tissue culture fluid. These observations of experimental animals dying from encephalitis led Culbertson et al. to predict a role for free-living amoebae as agents of human disease. Human cases of amoebic encephalitis were reported soon thereafter. The first cases which clearly established *Acanthamoebae* as causative agents of disease in humans were reported in the early 1970s with many more reports of various diseases following ever since (Dunand et al., 1997; Gulett et al., 1979; Illingworth & Cook 1998; Jones et al., 1975; Martinez et al., 1994).

Acanthamoeba spp. are among the most prevalent protozoa found in the environment. They are distributed worldwide and have been isolated from soil, dust, air, natural and treated water, seawater, swimming pools, sewage, sediments, air-conditioning units, drinking water treatment plants, bottled water, dental treatment units, hospitals and dialysis units, eyewash stations, and contact lenses and lens cases and as contaminants in bacterial, yeast, and mammalian cell cultures *Acanthamoeba* spp. also have been isolated from vegetation, from animals including fish, amphibia, reptiles, and mammals, from the nasal mucosa and throats of apparently healthy humans, from infected brain and lung tissue, from skin lesions of immunosuppressed patients, and from corneal tissue of patients with Acanthamoeba keratitis. It has been shown to live in domestic tap water pipelines especially in the cold water systems (Gray et al., 1995; Kilvington et al., 2004; Marciano-Cabral & Cabral, 2003; Radford et al., 1995).

The life cycle of *Acanthamoeba* consists of two stages: an actively feeding, dividing trophozoite and a dormant cyst. The trophozoite varies in size from 25 to 40 μm and feeds on bacteria, algae, and yeast in the environment but can also exist axenically on nutrients in liquid taken up through pinocytosis. A double-walled wrinkled cyst composed of an ectocyst and an endocyst ranges in size from 13 to 20 μm and varies from species to species. Cyst formation occurs under adverse environmental conditions such as food deprivation, desiccation, and changes in temperature and pH. Cysts are resistant to biocides, chlorination, and antibiotics and survive low temperatures (0 to 2°C). But treatment with Freon or methylene oxide or autoclaving destroys cysts. Excystment occurs when trophozoites emerge from the cyst under suitable environmental conditions. It was demonstrated that cysts retained viable amoebae for over 24 years after storage in water at 4°C (Khan, 2001; Marciano-Cabral & Cabral, 2003).

The cellular organization of *Acanthamoeba* has been studied using electron microscopy. Organelles typically found in higher eukaryotic cells have been identified in *Acanthamoebae.* They have a Golgi complex, smooth and rough endoplasmic reticula, free ribosomes, digestive vacuoles, mitochondria, and microtubules in *Acanthamoeba* trophozoites. A trilaminar plasma membrane was found to surround the cytoplasmic contents of the trophozoite. In addition, distinguishing features of the trophozoite were the presence of spiny surface projections called acanthopodia, a prominent contractile vacuole in the cytoplasm that controls the water content of the cell, and a nucleus with a large central nucleolus. Generally, the amoebae are uninucleated, although multinucleated cells are common when *Acanthamoeba* are maintained in suspension culture. Reproduction occurs by binary fission (Marciano-Cabral & Cabral, 2003).

Pathogenic Acanthamoeba exhibited higher numbers (above hundred) of acanthopodia as compared to non-pathogens (below twenty) (Khan, 2001). *Acanthamoeba* species can be assigned to three different groups on the basis of their cyst morphology. Later the complete gene sequence of nuclear small ribosomal subunit RNA was determined and using this approach, *Acanthamoeba* species was classified into 53 isolates on the basis of 12 rDNA

sequence types (RNA genotypes) designated typing units T1 to T12. Additional sequence types may exist. Sequences of either nuclear (RNA) or mitochondrial rRNA genes are suitable for classifying isolates. Current classification schemes integrate the morphological groups with the 12 sequence types (RNA genotypes) (T1 to T12) so that group I includes sequence types T7, T8, and T9, group II includes sequence types T3, T4, and T11, and group III includes sequence types T1, T2, T5, T6, T10, andT12. Studies in which clinical isolates have been identified based on sequence types have shown that the majority of strains causing keratitis belong to sequence type 4 (Marciano-Cabral & Cabral, 2003).
Amoebae have been reported to exhibit different capabilities for binding and internalizing different species of bacteria. Bacterium amoebae interactions may lead to the establishment of an endosymbiotic state or, alternatively, to destruction of either the bacterium or the amoeba. The role of *Acanthamoeba* spp. as reservoirs or vectors for human pathogens has been examined. The intracellular growth of bacteria in *Acanthamoeba* has been associated with enhanced survival of bacteria in the environment, increased resistance of bacteria to biocides, and increased bacterial virulence. Intracellular survival within the amoebae has been postulated as a mode by which bacteria survive in substrate-limiting environmental ecosystems. Intracellular growth of bacteria in amoebae apparently also affects the resistance of bacteria to antibiotics (Marciano-Cabral & Cabral, 2003).

1.2 Pathogenesis

Pathogenic and nonpathogenic strains of *Acanthamoebae* have already been isolated from the environment, but the pathogenesis of infection and the biochemical determinants of virulence are poorly understood. Temperature tolerance, growth rate, adherence properties, cytolytic products produced by amoebae, and immune evasion mechanisms appear to constitute important factors in their pathogenicity. The virulence of pathogenic amoebae wanes during continuous culture in axenic medium but can be restored by brain passage in mice. It has been proposed that virulence may be related to distinct physiological characteristics of a strain and not to a dependence on environmental conditions (Marciano-Cabral & Cabral, 2003).
Animal studies have confirmed the clinical impression that contact lenses are vectors for transmitting trophozoites to the corneal surface and facilitating trophozoite binding to the corneal epithelium. Adherence of trophozoites to cells followed by injury and invasion of tissue are thought to represent important steps in the establishment of infections. Clinical isolates of *A. polyphaga*, *A. castellanii*, and *A. culbertsoni* have been shown to attach to corneal epithelial cells through a process which involves binding to cell surface carbohydrate moieties. *A. castellanii* binds to mannose containing glycoproteins on the corneal epithelium through a 136-kDa mannose-binding protein on the amoeba surface. The adherence of *Acanthamoeba* to corneal epithelial cells can be inhibited by mannose and methylmannose pyranoside but not by other sugars (Clarke & Niederkorn, 2003; Hurt et al., 2003; Marciano-Cabral & Cabral, 2003). Glycolipids of corneal epithelium reactive with *Acanthamoeba* may also play a role in the pathogenesis of Acanthamoeba keratitis by mediating the adherence of the amoebae to the cornea. Gordon et al., using binding assays, reported that *Acanthamoeba* binds preferentially to collagen IV, laminin, and fibronectin (Gordon et al., 1993).
Following adherence to cells, invasion and extensive tissue destruction occur in the host. Human epithelial cells, stromal keratocytes, and stromal cell homogenates have been used in vitro as models of Acanthamoeba keratitis. Damage to cells and tissue is thought to occur by phagocytic processes and by cytotoxic substances released by amoebae. Exposure to

mannose induces Acanthamoeba trophozoites to produce a 133-kDa protease termed mannose-induced-protein (MIP) 133. MIP133 produces contact independent cytolysis of corneal epithelial cells in vitro. Corneal organ culture studies have shown that binding to mannose glycoproteins on the traumatized corneal epithelium induces trophozoites to release cytopathic factors (including MIP133) that facilitate corneal destruction and invasion. Activated MMPs degrade components of the basement membrane and the extracellular matrix, including types I and II collagens, fibronectin and laminin (Clarke & Niederkorn, 2006; Hurt et al., 2003). Acanthamoeba trophozoites use multiple proteases with nonspecific collagenolytic activity to penetrate and degrade the stroma; these include serine proteases, cysteine protease, an elastase and a metalloproteinase. In addition, there is evidence that a collagenolytic enzyme could have a role in the generation of the ring-like stromal infiltrates and corneal lesions that are characteristic of Acanthamoeba keratitis. Trophozoite adherence was followed by penetration, a process which appeared to involve both secretion of lytic enzymes and phagocytosis (Clarke & Niederkorn, 2006; Hurt et al., 2003).

1.3 Epidemiology, risk factors

Acanthamoeba spp. are among the most prevalent protozoa found in the environment. This spp. are worldwide and could been isolated from different sites so as soil, dust, air, natural and treated water, seawater, swimming pools, domestic tap water, drinking water, or even bottled water. The number of Acanthamoeba in a freshwater lake bottom can be 200-2100 amoeba/g. In the Potomac River for example there was one amoeba per 3.4 L water. The highest percentage of pathogens is during spring and fall (Nwachuku & Gerba, 2004). Acanthamoebae have been detected in tap water and in swimming pools. In Mexico amoebae were found in 13% of the water samples from faucets in private residences. In Egypt 2/50 tap water samples were contaminated. In Germany amoebae were found in 56% of hot water taps examined in hospitals. In England amoebae were isolated from bathroom and kitchen cold water taps. Amoebae may survive pool and spa disinfection (bromine, chlorine) procedures because of their resistant cyst stages. In 1977 *Acanthamoebae* were recovered in the water of 27 out of 30 public pools. Acanthamoeba has been isolated in swimming pools in Germany, Mexico and in Norway, temperature-tolerant strains of Acanthamoeba in spas in New Zealand and Spain. Acanthamoeba was isolated from bottled water also in Mexico. Acanthamoeba cyst can be isolated from air, dust, air conditioner, cooling towers (Kilvington et al., 2004; Nwachuku & Gerba, 2004). Acanthamoebic keratitis first reported by Nagington et al. (Nagington et al., 1974) in Great Britain and by Jones et al. Jones et al., 1975) in the United States is a painful progressive sight-threatening corneal disease. Since acanthamoebic keratitis is not a reportable disease, the true incidence is not known. Published works suggest an incidence rate of 0.58-0.71 cases/1.000.000 in the general population, and 1.65-2.01/1.000.000 among contact lens wearers (Nwachuku & Gerba, 2004). The given incidence among contact lens wearers is 3-5/1.000.000 in Holland, and 33/1.000.000 in Hong Kong (Seal, 2003). Three recent multi centre Questionnaire Reporting Surveys of Acanthamoeba keratitis were conducted in England within the past twenty years. The first in 1992–96 gave an incidence rate of 0.25 per 10 000 contact lens wearers (CLW). The second and third surveys in England and Wales carried out in 1997–99 with one case in 47 620 CLW (or 0.21 per 10 000) and in 1998–99 with one case in 555 CLW (or 0.18 per 10 000) found that 80% of all infections were manifest in lens wearers, with 88% using hydrogel lenses and 12% rigid lenses The incidence of acanthamoeba keratitis with gas permeable and rigid contact lenses is much lower than with soft hydrogel CL (Seal,

2003). In non contact lens wearers history of trauma in a garden is a risk factor (Radford et al., 1998).

Patient ages range from 4 to 64 years, with a mean age of 30 years, with no difference in genders (Radford et al., 1998; Sharma et al., 2000). Infection usually affects only one eye, although the infection is occasionally bilateral (Illingworth & Cook, 1998; Parthasarathy et al., 2007; Radford et al., 1998; Wilhelmus et al., 2008). Among non contact lens wearers trauma and exposure to contaminated water have been identified as major risk factors (Chynn et al., 1995; Sharma et al., 2000). Multivariable analysis showed that this is largely attributable to a lack of disinfection, the use of non-sterile saline, and the use of chlorine based disinfection rather than alternative chemical systems (Radford et al., 1995). Many CL users are still contaminating their contact lenses with tap water either directly (showering, face washing, handling with wet hands) or by using water to rinse their storage case (Radford et al., 2002; Seal et al., 1999). Disposable soft contact lenses seem to be a risk factor for contact lens induced keratitis. 89% of the patients with keratitis used this type of contact lens (Dejaco-Ruhswurm et al., 2001). It was shown that adherence of amoeba to the lens was higher among disposable contact lenses (etafilcon A) than among the conventional lenses (polymacon) (Beattie et al., 2003, Lema et al., 2001). Attachment of Acanthamoeba was affected significantly by lens material type ($P<0.001$), with higher numbers of trophozoites attaching to the first-generation lotrafilcon A silicone hydrogel lens, compared with the second-generation galyfilcon A lens and the conventional hydrogel lens. Patient wear and the presence of a bacterial biofilm had no significant effect on the attachment to the lotrafilcon A lens but did significantly increase attachment to the galyfilcon A and the etafilcon A ($P = 0.009$) lenses. If exposed to Acanthamoeba (e.g., when showering or swimming, through non-continuous wear and ineffective lens care regimes), first-generation silicone hydrogel lenses may promote a greater risk of Acanthamoeba infection due to the enhanced attachment characteristics of this lens material (Beattie et al., 2006).

An initial coinfection occurs, with the bacteria providing an additional food source for the amoebae. The presence of bacterial biofilm may also affect amoebal sensitivity to disinfectants (Illingworth & Cook, 1998).

Trophozoite and cyst adherence of two acanthamoeba keratitis strains to four types of unworn soft contact lens and their removal by cleaning agents were studied. Greater adherence of the trophozoites compared with the cysts was recorded. Trophozoites adhered in greater numbers to type I lenses (poly2-hydroxyethyl methacrylate), with no differences between type II (lidofilcon A), III (bufilcon A) and IV (etafilcon A) lenses. Adherence of the other trophozoites to type II lenses was lower compared with their adherence to the other lenses. Cysts of both strains showed greater adherence to type I and III lenses. Recommended cleaning procedures using three commercial solutions were effective in removing Acanthamoeba from the lenses (Kilvington, 1993).

1.4 Clinical symptoms

The clinical picture of acanthamoeba keratitis is remarkable for its varied manifestations, although these often seem to occur in a recognizable sequence. Most patients complain of symptoms of photophobia, pain, and tearing. The pain in acanthamoeba keratitis may be particularly severe, seemingly disproportionate to the signs, although the absence of severe pain does not preclude the diagnosis. Rarely, there may be an apparent precipitating event, such as an injury to the eye, swimming while wearing lenses, or insertion of a non-sterile lens. Symptoms may continue uninterrupted from the time of an injury, sometimes with apparent failure of a corneal abrasion to heal, or rarely, there may be a delay of up to 2 weeks before the onset of symptoms. The earliest signs may be non-specific and may take the form of epithelial micro erosions, irregularities, opacities or microcystic oedema, often with patchy anterior stromal infiltrates. There may be no fluorescein staining at the onset. Commonly, there is a dendriform keratitis that is often initially treated as herpes simplex infection. Limbitis (limbal hyperaemia and oedema) is a very frequent finding in both early as well as late stages of the disease. A pattern of perineural infiltrates that occurs in a radial distribution (radial keratoneuritis) is virtually pathognomic for acanthamoeba keratitis. A ring infiltrate, usually with an overlying epithelial defect is commonly seen. Although initially the epithelium within the ring may be intact, in longstanding cases a central defect, which is often associated with stromal thinning, may occur. The ring may be incomplete, or occasionally it is double and concentric. The inflammation may involve the sclera, evidence of direct scleral invasion by amoebae has often been elusive, leading to the conclusion that scleritis is a secondary immunologic reaction. Posterior segment signs are rare, although occasional reports of optic nerve oedema, optic neuropathy and optic atrophy, retinal detachment, choroidal inflammation, and formation of a macular scar exist. Contra lateral chorioretinitis has also been observed. In up to 20% of cases cataract may occur, although this appears to be associated with severe or prolonged inflammation, and use of topical corticosteroids. Glaucoma is commonly reported, particularly in advanced stages (Illingworth & Cook, 1998; Radford et al., 1998; Reinhard & Sundmacher, 2000).

1.5 Diagnosis

The importance of early diagnosis cannot be overemphasized. We have to consider acanthamoeba keratitis when symptoms associated with trauma especially involving vegetable matter or exposure to contaminated water, such as lake -, sea-, or spring water are mentioned. Early diagnosis is essential to ensure a good prognosis. If effective therapy is delayed for 3 or more weeks the prognosis will deteriorate. Acanthamoeba keratitis should be considered in any case of corneal trauma complicated by exposure to soil or contaminated water, and in all CL wearers (Dart et al., 2009). We also have to question the patients about this during the history taking.

Acanthamoebic keratitis has to be differentiated from bacterial or fungal or herpes simplex virus (HSV) keratitis. In addition, the disease must be considered when there is a failure to respond to first-line therapy for bacterial or herpes simplex virus keratitis, even when there has been a positive culture for another organism, because 10% to 23% of cases of Acanthamoeba keratitis may be polymicrobial or co-infected. Perineural and/or ring infiltrates are characteristic clinical signs of the disease (Dart et al., 2009; Marciano-Cabral & Cabral, 2003; Radford et al., 1998).

Diagnosis may be achieved by using different methods, including non invasive confocal microscopy which is the preferred diagnostic technique in some centres, with sensitivity and specificity exceeding 90% (Dart et al., 2009). Another quick method is staining corneal scrapings with acridine orange, which reveal yellow-to-orange polygonal, cystic structures consistent with the appearance of *Acanthamoeba* among inflammatory cells and the corneal epithelial cells (Hahn et al., 1998). An additional advantage of the method is that no special solutions and staining techniques are required. A definitive diagnosis of Acanthamoeba keratitis can only be made on the basis of culture or histology, or by the identification of the presence of amoebic DNA with PCR (Dart et al., 2009). Corneal scrapes or corneal biopsy specimens are used for culture or for the identification of cysts or trophozoites in stained tissue sections. For culture, material from a corneal scrape can be placed onto no nutrient agar containing *E. coli*. It should be incubated at 28 to 35°C and held for an extended interval (10 days or more to ensure time for excystation) because some species of *Acanthamoeba* do not grow well at 35°C or above. However, corneal scrapes may contain bacteria or yeast, which can confuse the diagnosis. Corneal biopsy has been suggested when repeated cultures of corneal scrapings are negative (Illingworth & Cook, 1998; Marciano-Cabral & Cabral, 2003). For a cytological diagnosis, various staining methods can be employed. The indirect immunofluorescent-antibody assay has been used to detect amoebae in corneal scrapings or in biopsy tissue. Calcofluor white, a chemo fluorescent dye with an affinity for the polysaccharide polymers of amoebic cysts, has been used to identify amoebic cysts in corneal tissue. Calcofluor white stains amoebic cyst walls bright apple green and this effect can be enhanced by prolonging the staining period. Evans blue is used to counter stain the background. Trophozoites and cysts in paraffin-embedded tissues can also be rapidly and differentially stained with calcofluor white (Marciano-Cabral & Cabral, 2003). For the rapid and sensitive identification of Acanthamoeba at the genus level, a polymerase chain reaction (PCR)-based method can be used. For typing *Acanthamoeba* isolates a restriction fragment length polymorphisms (RFLPs) is useful (Khan et al., 2001; Kilvington et al., 2004).

1.6 Treatment

The goals of medical therapy in Acanthamoeba keratitis include the eradication of viable cysts and trophozoites and rapid resolution of the associated inflammatory response.

1.6.1 Medical treatment

There is no single drug capable of eliminating the infection therefore drug combinations have been suggested as a treatment regimen. Several drugs are known to be amoebicid and cysticid. There are currently no drugs that are effective as monoterapy in Acanthamoeba keratitis, so combinations are suggested. Acanthamoeba trophozoites are sensitive to most available chemotherapeutic agents (antibiotics, antiseptics, antifungals, antiprotozoals including metronidazole, antiviral, and antineoplastic agents). However, persistent infection is related to the presence of *Acanthamoeba* cysts, against which very few of these agents have any effect and only agents that are cysticidal in vitro against cysts can be expected to be effective as therapy. The diamidines and biguanides are currently the most effective cysticidal antiamoebics in vitro and their use is supported by substantial case series. Metronidazole (Flagyl; Pfizer Inc, New York, New York, USA) has been used for several cases in one series, but has proved to have no effect in vitro. For these reasons topical therapy with biguanides with or without the addition of diamidines is currently the mainstay of treatment for Acanthamoeba keratitis (Bacon et al., 1993; Dart et al., 2009; Illingworth et al., 1995; Illingworth & Cook, 1998; McCellan et al., 2001; Seal, 2003).

Biguanides: The two biguanides that are in use are polyhexamethylene biguanide (PHMB) 0.02% to 0.06% (200 to 600 g/ml) and chlorhexidine 0.02% to 0.2% (200 to 2000 g/ml). The biguanides interact with the cytoplasmic membrane, resulting in loss of cellular components and inhibition of respiratory enzymes. Both drugs have been effective clinically as primary therapy, as well as in cases where other agents have failed. Clinically, corneal epithelial toxicity has been minimal for both chlorhexidine 0.02% and PHMB 0.02%. Biguanides can be used as first-line treatment for Acanthamoeba keratitis either alone or in combination with diamidines, with which there may be a synergistic or additive effect (Bacon et al., 1993; Dart et al., 2009; Illingworth et al., 1995; Illingworth & Cook, 1998; McCellan et al., 2001; Seal, 2003).

Diamidines. Available diamidines include propamidine isethionate 0.1% (1000 g/ml) and hexamidine 0.1% (1000 g/ml); these are licensed as antibacterials in some European countries. The antimicrobial effects of the diamidines result from the cationic surface-active properties inducing structural membrane changes affecting cell permeability. When these molecules penetrate into the amoebic cytoplasm, denaturation of cytoplasmic proteins and enzymes occurs. Propamidine and hexamidine have been effective clinically against both the trophozoite and cyst forms of *Acanthamoeba.* Clinically, the diamidines are well tolerated by ocular tissues, although prolonged treatment with propamidine may lead to toxic keratopathy (Bacon et al., 1993; Dart et al., 2009; Illingworth et al., 1995; Illingworth & Cook, 1998; McCellan et al., 2001; Seal, 2003).

Although neomycin has been widely used, it is ineffective against cysts in vitro. In addition, like all aminoglycosides it is toxic to the corneal epithelium and can often result in indolent corneal ulceration that may be incorrectly attributed to disease activity, nevertheless it is effective for the bacterial co-infection. Povidon-Iodine (Betadine) is amoebicid and cysticid generally, however it can be used in 0.5% concentrate as well (Bacon et al., 1993; Dart et al., 2009; Illingworth et al., 1995; Illingworth & Cook, 1998; McCellan et al., 2001; Seal, 2003).

Topical corticosteroids. The role of steroids is controversial, but we believe that topical corticosteroids can have an important and beneficial role in the management of some cases of Acanthamoeba keratitis. The dead cysts persist in the corneal stroma and remain antigenic. This can give rise to a serious inflammatory reaction. Steroid treatment is unnecessary in most cases diagnosed early, which usually respond rapidly to antiamoebic drugs. However, persisting inflammation (anterior scleritis, severe pain, indolent ulcers, corneal inflammation, and anterior chamber inflammation) may respond dramatically to the addition of even low-potency topical steroid therapy, e.g. prednisolone 0.5%, or dexamethasone 0.1% 4 times daily. Clinicians should be careful to avoid use of corticosteroids if possible because they suppress the activity of the macrophage, which is the 'scavenger' phagocytic cell responsible for host immunity to Acanthamoeba. Use of nonsteroidal anti-inflammatory drugs, particularly flurbiprofen, is encouraged and also acts as both an analgesic and a mydriatic. When attendant to the inflammation secondary glaucoma appears, anti-glaucomatic drops are used. Pupil dilatators are also used for moving the pupil (Bacon et al., 1993; Dart et al., 2009; Illingworth et al., 1995; Illingworth & Cook, 1998; McCellan et al., 2001; Seal, 2003).

1.6.2 Surgical treatment

With respect to the severity of the disease as well as the complications accompanying it there is a range of surgical methods to choose from.

Corneal abrasion or debridement of the affected area of corneal epithelium may be successful if performed at an early stage. Repeated debridement is used in some centres to improve drug penetration (Dart et al., 2009; Illingworth & Cook, 1998; Reinhard & Sundmacher, 2000).

Cryosurgery may be valuable in treating Acanthamoeba keratitis cases. Cryocoagulation to the ring infiltrate and central cornea breaks the infected cells and cyst walls (Amoils & Heney, 1999; Reinhard & Sundmacher, 2000).

Deep lamellar keratectomy with a conjunctival flap is a suitable approach to help control the infection and to help relieve pain in patients with advanced Acanthamoeba keratitis (Cremon et al., 2002; Parthasarathy & Tan, 2007).

Instead of conjunctiva, *amniotic membrane* is usable. This suggests that amnion cells in amniotic membrane release proteinase inhibitors and that stromal matrix selectively provide adhesion molecules for polymorphonuclear cells (Kim et al., 2000). Amniotic membrane transplantation may be a safe and effective treatment of severe Acanthamoeba keratitis, particularly during the inflammation phase. It may permit penetrating keratoplasty to be delayed (Bourcier et al., 2004).
The role of *keratoplasty* is now largely restricted to the visual rehabilitation of eyes in which a medical cure has been achieved. In advanced cases corneal transplantation may be necessary. Because of use of antiamoebal agents, penetrating keratoplasty is now usually unnecessary in the acute phase unless the cornea has become very thin, with consequent risk of perforation (Bacon et al, 1993; Dart et al., 2009; Illingworth & Cook, 1998; Reinhard & Sundmacher, 2000).
Deep lamellar keratoplasty (DLK) with total removal of infected stromal tissue may be performed in medically unresponsive cases of Acanthamoeba keratitis. Advantages of DLK in infectious keratitis include less risk of intraocular entry of infectious organisms at the time of surgery and the potential for improved graft survival rates caused by less endothelial rejection and failure. In patients with severe disease involving the visual axis, earlier surgery with DLK would allow debulking of the organisms as well as preservation of autogenous endothelial cell function (Parthasarathy & Tan, 2007; Por et al., 2009; Taenaka et al., 2007).
In some cases enucleation or evisceration is needed, because of inflammation, infection or secundary glaucoma (Bacon et al., 1993; Radford et al., 1998; Reinhard & Sundmacher, 2000).

2. Mean headings

2.1 Patients, methods and results

Patients' features and clinical data are summarised in Table 1.

pati-ent	age	sex	time till diagnosis	BCVA	diagnosis	clinical features	medical treatment	keratoplasty	surgical treatment	BCVA at latest follow up
1.	25	female	3 days	0.01	corneal scrape	corneal ulcus	dimopropamide +neomycine +ciprofloxacin +diclofenac +cyclopentholat	after 2 years urgency keratoplasty (7.75/8.0 mm) because descemetocele	aspiration lentis, scleral buckling, vitrectomy	light perceptio n
2.	26	female	2 weeks	0.01	clinical findings	central ring-infiltratio n	dimopropamide +PHMB +neomycine +ciprofloxacin +prednisolon +atropin +cyclopentholat	after 3 month proposed keratoplasty (7.0/7.25 mm)		0.7
3.	41	female	4 weeks	0.03	histology	central corneal ulcus, hypopyon	dimopropamide +PHMB +neomycine +ciprofloxacin +diclofenac	after 4 month proposed keratoplasty (7.0/7.75 mm)		1.0

patient	age	sex	time till diagnosis	BCVA	diagnosis	clinical features	medical treatment	keratoplasty	surgical treatment	BCVA at latest follow up
4.	23	male	4 weeks	0.02	corneal scrape	central corneal abscess	dimopropamide +PHMB +neomycine +ciprofloxacin +diclofenac +timolol	after 1 month urgency keratoplasty (7.0/7.5 mm)		light perception
5.	33	female	4 weeks	0.02	histology	central infiltration	dimopropamide +neomycine +fluorometholon +cyclopentholat	after 6 month urgency keratoplasty (7.5/7.5 mm)	corneal abrasion, phaco-emulsifikation +IOL	0.9
6.	65	female	2 months	0.15	clinical findings	central ring-infiltration	dimopropamide +PHMB +neomycine +ciprofloxacin +diclofenac	after 2 years urgency keratoplasty (7.7/8.25 mm)	ECCE+PCL+ trabeculectomy after 1 year	light perception

Table 1. Clinical data of our patients (BCVA=best corrected visual acuity)

2.1.1 Demographics

Between 2001 and 2006 we treated 11 patients with Acanthamoeba keratitis. The mean age of the patients was 30.2 years (16-65). The eight female and three male patients were all soft contact lens wearers. The right eye was affected in six and the left in five cases. 82% of the infections occurred in the summer period between June and September. The appropriate diagnosis of Acanthamoeba keratitis took 3 days to 2 months. Beside long-lasting conservative treatment perforating keratoplasty was performed in six cases. In the following we discuss these patients in details.

2.1.2 Risk factors

The infection was caused by poor and improper contact lens hygiene in each and every case. All lenses involved were hydrogel soft lenses: 1 daily, 4 monthly and 1 yearly disposable. None of the lenses have been applied for extended or continuous wear. Two patients rinsed the lenses in tap water, 4 patients went to swim in them. The half of the patients got the lenses from opticians, the other half from ophthalmologists.

2.1.3 Clinical findings and diagnosis

Significant visual decrease (0.15-0.01) was seen in almost all cases. Slit lamp examination showed corneal infiltration in 2 cases, ring infiltration (Fig. 1. and 2.) in 3 cases and corneal abscess in 1 case. The diagnosis was based on corneal scraping in 2 cases, on histology in 2 cases, and on clinical findings in 2 cases.

2.1.4 Medical treatment

Treatment started with antiamoebic agents in all patients: dibromopropamide or propamidin and polihexamethilen biguanidine was administerd hourly in the first week, and then 5 times/day for at least 6 months. All patients were administered antibiotic drops 5 times a day for 2 weeks. Two patients had to use antiglaucomatic drops because of secondary glaucoma. We used steroid or non-steroid agents against the inflammation in seven cases.

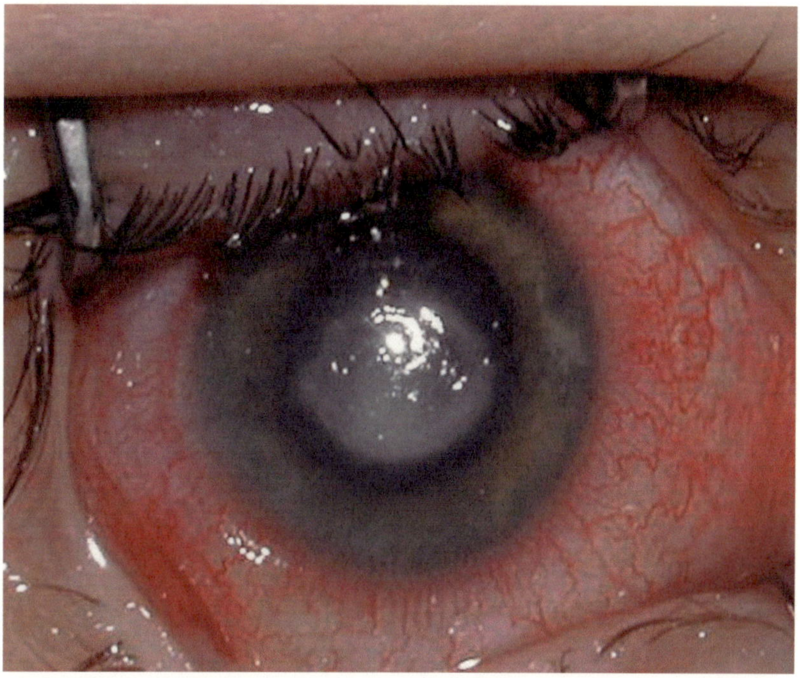

Fig. 1. Anterior segment of patient N° 5 before keratoplasty with corneal abscess

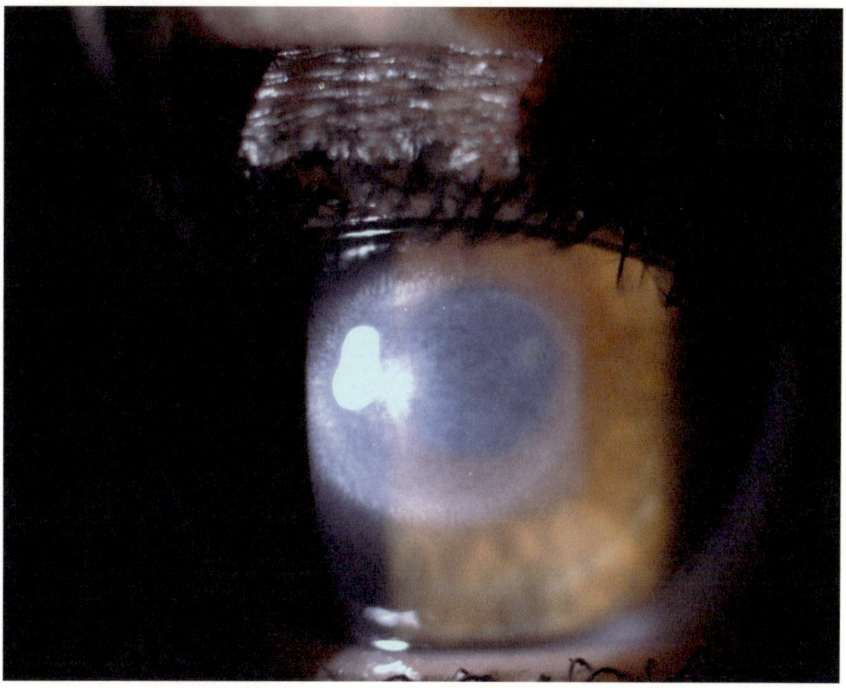

Fig. 2. Corneal scar of patient N° 2 before optical keratoplasty

2.1.5 Indications for surgical intervention

In one case we performed corneal abrasion, but as it proved ineffective we followed it up with perforating keratoplasty.

Perforating keratoplasty was performed in six cases. In four cases keratoplasty was performed as an emergency to save the eyeball (because of descemetocele), in two cases the operations were scheduled for visual rehabilitation. The emergency cases were the "late diagnostic" cases.

Shape and size of keratoplasty and surgical techniques: All keratoplasties were perforating (penetrating), and central. All surgical procedures were done by two experienced surgeons. All cases were performed under retrobulbar anaesthesia. The trephination was performed with modified Geuder trephines for the host cornea from the epithelial side, and the graft from the endothelial side. Donor corneas were from the Eye Bank of our department. Only grafts with an endothelial cell count above 2000 cells/mm^2 were used. The mean graft diameter was 7.7 mm (range 7.25 to 8.25 mm), with an average over sizing of 0.5 mm. Graft fixation was performed in all cases with running nylon 10/0 sutures. (Fig. 3.,4.)

2.1.6 Postoperative management

Topical antibiotic and steroid drops were used five times a day for 6 weeks, then only steroid drops for 6 months. Anti amoebatic drops 5 times/day for at least six months.

2.1.7 Complications

We have had no intraoperative complications. Postoperative glaucoma appeared in 2 cases, in one case trabeculectomy was performed. In 3 cases cataract operation was necessary after some months. In one case retinal detachment developed and therefore scleral buckling operation was needed.

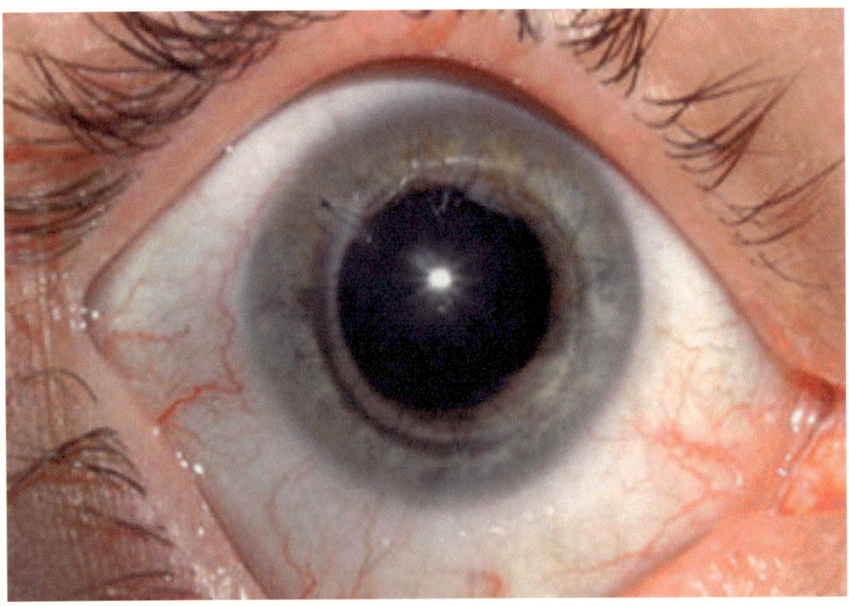

Fig. 3. Postoperative status of perforated keratoplasty of patient N° 5.

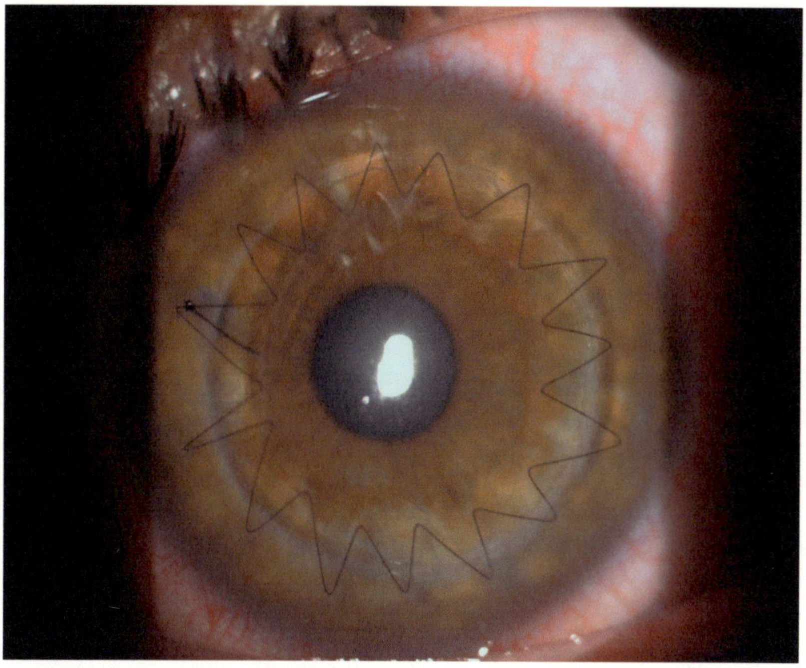

Fig. 4. Early postoperative status of patient Nº 2.

2.1.8 Graft clarity and visual acuity

At the last follow up visit the visual acuity was 0.43. In 3 cases it was only light perception, but the other 3 patients had very good visual acuity (0.7-1.0).

In the emergency cases the visual acuity was much worse (light perception in 3 cases and 0.9 in one case), then in the proposed cases (0.7 and 1.0). In 5 cases the cornea graft was clear, rejection and decompensation developed only in one case.

2.2 Corneal graft surgery/keratoplasty

2.2.1 Emergency keratoplasty

Emergency keratoplasty or keratoplasty à chaud is often the only possible intervention to prevent complete and irreversible vision loss in patients with severe corneal disorders. The main indications for this urgent surgical procedure are corneal perforations or imminent perforations, maintaining the integrity of the globe, as well as persisting infectious keratitis. Due to acute inflammation of the anterior ocular segment, emergency keratoplasty is supposed to have a worse outcome and more postoperative complications especially more immune reactions than scheduled keratoplasty. Keratoplasty for management of the acute complications of Acanthamoeba keratitis has with few exceptions in small numbers of patients (Illingworth & Cook, 1998; Nguyen et al., 2010; Maier et al., 2007; Shi et al., 2009), generally been reported to have poor results. Graft failure due to recurrent infection is common when keratoplasty is performed in an inflamed eye. In most cases, however, keratoplasty has been successful in maintaining the integrity of the globe, and a second procedure has often resulted in a good visual outcome (Illingworth & Cook, 1998; Maier et al., 2007).

Since the introduction of the biguanides as medical therapy, PK has not been recommended as a treatment for the elimination of organisms; emergency keratoplasty should therefore be reserved as a treatment for corneal perforation, imminent perforation and fulminant corneal abscess. Many of these eyes will be severely inflamed with uncontrolled scleritis and limbitis, which should be treated before surgery with systemic immunsuppression using prednisolone (0.5 to 1 mg/kg/day) and/or cyclosporine (3 to 7.5 mg/kg/day), which is tapered as inflammation is controlled in the post graft period (Dart et al. 2009; Maier et al., 2007). Performing PK before scleral or peripheral corneal extension can minimize the risk of recurrence and poor outcome (Nguyen et al., 2010; Tanhehco & Colby, 2010).

2.2.2 Therapeutic/optical keratoplasty

Several authors (Awwad et al., 2005; Por et al., 2009) recommend observing for at least 3 months of clinical inactivity after completion of antiamoebic therapy before attempting PK. Most recently, Kitzmann et al. (Kitzmann et al., 2009) compared outcomes of 22 eyes with Acanthamoeba keratitis undergoing emergency penetrating or anterior lamellar keratoplasty and 9 eyes undergoing optical penetrating or anterior lamellar keratoplasty. Although all eyes ultimately achieved microbiological cure, there was a 41% recurrence rate of Acanthamoeba keratitis after emergency keratoplasty compared with 22% recurrence rate after optical keratoplasty. The Kaplan–Meier graft survival was 37.5% (95% confidence interval, 16.8–58.4) at 5 years in the therapeutic group compared with 100% in the optical group. Shi et al. (Shi et al., 2009) reported 28% recurrence after emergency PK. For acanthamoeba keratitis, Ficker et al. (Ficker et al., 1993) found that clear graft survival was only 20% if penetrating keratoplasty was performed during the acute, inflamed state of the disease compared to 100% clear graft survival when penetrating keratoplasty was performed in a quiet state of the disease. The reason for the difference compared to other results might possibly be differences in case selection at the time of diagnosis, preoperative treatment and the time point of the decision for emergency keratoplasty seem to be most important for the outcome of the graft (Maier et al., 2007). Dart et al. (Dart et al., 2009) present cases, when therapeutic keratoplasty is rarely used but lamellar or PK to improve vision is carried out in patients with scarred corneas and/or irregular astigmatism. The outcome of corneal transplantation is good in this group of patients. Exacerbations of scleritis and limbitis may occur following graft surgery in these eyes and may need to be treated with systemic anti-inflammatory treatment (Dart et al., 2009). Quian et al. (Qian et al., 2010) performed 8 optical perforating keratoplasty after at least 4 months medical treatment, with great success. Awwad et al. (Awwad et al., 2005) published an article about 13 eyes which underwent optical PK for visual rehabilitation after acanthamoeba keratitis. They mean that PK for visual restoration after resolution of *Acanthamoeba* keratitis in quiet eyes that are judged cyst-free by preoperative confocal microscopy appears to have an excellent long-term prognosis. Waiting at least 3 months after the discontinuation of medical therapy also appears helpful to rule out latent infection because of cyst reactivation and to allow the active inflammation to cease.
The success of keratoplasty in the literature are summarised in Table 2.

2.2.3 Donor size

The extent of the infected corneal tissue cannot be identified and should be assumed to include the entire cornea so that, unlike grafts for other corneal infections, which should be large enough to remove all contaminated tissue, the graft for Acanthamoeba keratitis should

author	year	total	acute	success %	optical	success %
Kitzmann	2009	30	22	45.5	8	100
Nguyen	2010	9	9	100		
Ficker	1993	13	7	20	6	100
Maier	2007	13	13	73		
Kashiwabuchi	2008	32	32	43.8		
Awwad	2005	13			13	100
Tanhehco	2010	8	8	50		
Qian	2010	8			8	100
Por	2009	15	12		3	
Illengworth	1995	9	9	100		
Bacon	1993	34	21	35	13	69
Radford	1998	31				
Sharma	2000	3	3	0		

Table 2. Success rate of keratoplasty

be kept to the minimum size required to excise all ulcerated and necrotic tissue, retaining clinically healthy (but usually subclinically infected) tissue. This is because of the risk of rejection with large grafts and because repeating grafting may be needed as a result of recurrence; a further graft represents a new food source for the organism and can be used to attract residual amoebae. Recurrence of disease in a graft was frequent in the first 2 weeks after surgery when keratoplasty was performed in an inflamed eye before the introduction of biguanides; it typically involved the donor periphery, usually without clinical involvement of the host. Late recurrences, several months after surgery, may also occur. The use of large grafts worsens the prognosis because it increases the chances of an immune response to the graft. Furthermore, the use of a large graft indicates a more severe preoperative infection (Ficker et al., 1993).

Host trephination size ranged from 7 to 11 mm depending on the extent of the corneal infiltration. The trephination should be performed beyond the clinical areas of infiltrate, including satellite lesions. Confocal microscopy can be used to outline the extent of involvement or the size of the trephination (Kashiwabuchiet al., 2008; Nguyen et al., 2010).

Meier et al. reported about a trend toward improved clear graft survival and fewer immune reactions following emergency keratoplasty using smaller grafts (≤8.00 mm) (Awwad et al., 2005; Maier et al., 2007).

Ideally, a corneal scar should be debulked as much as possible because residual cysts might still be present and might lead potentially to a recurrence of the disease when exposed to topical corticosteroids after PK. In those cases, rather than jeopardizing graft survival by trephining a large donor button (sizes of 9 mm and beyond), we suggest waiting for a longer period of time after the discontinuation of medical treatment, with repetitive confocal examination when available, before committing the patient to surgery (Awwad et al, 2005).

3. Prevention

Acanthamoeba keratitis is a potentially blinding condition of the eye, and any steps toward prevention of this disease are encouraged. It is recommended contact lens wearers to use daily disposable contact lenses to eliminate the contact lens case as a reservoir for Acanthamoeba. If daily disposable contact lens can not be used, then hydrogen peroxide cleaning solutions are preferred over the more common multipurpose solutions because of the increased efficacy of hydrogen peroxide against Acanthamoeba cysts. Planned replacement of contact lens storage cases may also help reduce contamination. It is important for eye care professionals not only to emphasize proper contact lens wear and hygiene in the prevention of infectious keratitis but also to maintain a high clinical suspicion for Acanthamoeba keratitis because an early diagnosis may lead to a better visual outcome (Tanhehco & Colby, 2010). The use of surfactant cleaner has been shown to be an effective way of removing Acanthamoeba trophozoites and cysts (Kilvington, 1993). In the light of these findings further research into the types of disinfectant used by patients with Acanthamoeba keratitis is required, with a view to calculating the relative risks of different lens type and disinfectant combinations. This series also show the importance of the fact that contact lens practitioners should ensure at the time of prescribing lenses that patients have understood all the disinfectant procedures (Illingworth et al., 1995). Gray et al. suggest leaving contact lens case open to dry air after heat disinfection. If hydrogen peroxide disinfection is the preferred solution, one has to use a two step hydrogen peroxide system. It is necessary to call one's attention to wash hands properly before handling contact lens cases and what is more important is to avoid homemade saline. The contact lens case should be replaced regularly. Nowadays the use of more frequently disposable contact lenses is highly recommended (Gray et al., 1995). Also the rub and rinse step should be mentioned as the critical part of the disinfection that may reduce significantly the microbiological load (Shih et al., 1985). Detailed education of contact lens wearers concerning of the entire disinfection procedure could reduce the incidence of Acanthamoeba keratitis further on. There is a persistent need to educate contact lens wearers continuously about the possible risk factors of Acanthamoeba keratitis, and since the frequency of Acanthamoeba keratitis appears to be largely determined by the ever changing trends in contact lens use, continued monitoring is indicated (Radford et al., 1998). All of the eye care practitioners have to call attention of all contact lens users to aware the wearing of soft contact lenses in case of swimming so as to reduce the number of patients with Acanthamoeba keratitis (Kaji et al., 2005; Kettesy et al., 2010). If even a soft contact lens wearer wants to swim, then daily disposable contact lens and swimming spectacles should be used.

4. Conclusion

Acanthamoebic keratitis, first reported by Nagington et al. in Great Britain and by Jones et al. in the United States, is a painful progressive sight-threatening corneal disease. The infection is a rather frequently occurring disease all over the world which can still cause serious or even total loss of vision despite improved diagnostic and therapeutic options. *Acanthamoeba* spp. are among the most prevalent protozoa found in the environment. They are distributed worldwide and have been isolated from soil, dust, air, natural and treated water, seawater, swimming pools, sewage, sediments, air-conditioning units, drinking water treatment plants, bottled water, dental treatment units, hospitals and dialysis units, eyewash stations, and contact lenses and lens cases and as contaminants in bacterial, yeast, and mammalian cells. It mainly affects contact lens wearers with poor hygiene. In non contact lens wearers history of trauma in a garden is a risk factor. Patients' ages range from 4 to 64 years, with a mean age of 30 years, with no difference in genders. Infection usually affects only one eye, although it is occasionally bilateral. Most patients complain of symptoms of photophobia, pain, and tearing. The earliest signs may be non-specific and may take the form of epithelial micro erosions, irregularities, opacities or microcystic oedema, often with patchy anterior stromal infiltrates. There may be no fluorescein staining at the onset. Commonly, there is a dendriform keratitis that is often initially treated as herpes simplex infection. A ring infiltrate, usually with an overlying epithelial defect, is commonly seen. The ring may be incomplete, or occasionally it is double and concentric. The importance of early diagnosis cannot be overemphasized. We have to consider Acanthamoeba keratitis when symptoms associated with trauma especially involving vegetable matter or exposure to contaminated water, such as lake-, sea-, or spring water are mentioned. Acanthamoebic keratitis has to be differentiated from bacterial or fungal or herpes simplex virus keratitis. Diagnosis may be achieved by using different methods, including non invasive confocal microscopy, staining corneal scrapings with acridine orange, corneal scrapes or corneal biopsy specimens onto no nutrient agar containing *E. coli.,* cytological various staining methods, like indirect immunofluorescent-antibody assay, polymerase chain reaction (PCR)-based method. The goals of medical therapy in Acanthamoeba keratitis include the eradication of viable cysts and trophozoites and rapid resolution of the associated inflammatory response. There is no single drug capable of eliminating the infection therefore drug combinations have been suggested as a treatment regimen. There are currently no drugs that are effective as monotherapy in Acanthamoeba keratitis, hence combinations are suggested. Acanthamoeba trophozoites are sensitive to most available chemotherapeutic agents (antibiotics, antiseptics, antifungals, antiprotozoals including metronidazole, antiviral, and antineoplastic agents). The diamidines and biguanides are currently the most effective cysticidal antiamoebics. With respect to the severity of the disease as well as the complications accompanying it there is a range of surgical methods to choose from. Corneal abrasion, cryosurgery, deep lamellar keratectomy with a conjunctival flap, amnion membrane transplantation, keratoplasty, deep lamellar keratoplasty. In some cases enucleation or evisceration is needed, because of severe inflammation, infection or secondary glaucoma. Antiamoebic therapy should be used before surgery and be continued postoperatively using drugs and doses that will minimize or avoid signs of toxicity. PHMB 0.02% has low clinical toxicity in most patients and is clinically less than that with either of the diamidines. We use PHMB 0.02% 6 to 8 times daily immediately after surgery, with an adequate level of topical steroid to control inflammation. This should be continued for at least 3 weeks while results of culture of the host keratectomy specimen are awaited. If viable organisms are cultured it is prudent to continue antiamoebic therapy 4 times daily while high-doses of steroids are needed usually for 6 months after surgery, as recurrent Acanthamoeba keratitis has occurred up to 3 months after an initially successful transplant. If culture of the excised host cornea is negative after 3 weeks we assume that most viable amoebae have been treated, and the topical antiamoebic therapy is reduced to 4 times daily and stopped after 1 month.

Between 2001 and 2006 we treated 11 patients with Acanthamoeba keratitis. The patients were all soft contact lens wearers. The right eye was affected in six and the left in five cases. 82% of the infections occurred in the summer period between June and September. Beside long-lasting conservative treatment perforating keratoplasty was performed nearly in half of the cases.

In every case the infection was caused by poor and improper contact lens hygiene. All lenses involved were hydrogel soft lenses: 1 daily, 4 monthly and 1 yearly disposable. None of the lenses were extended or continuous wear. The half of the patients got the lenses from opticians, the other half from ophthalmologists.

Significant visual decrease was seen in almost all cases. Slit lamp examination showed corneal infiltration in 2 cases, ring infiltration (Fig. 1. and 2.) in 3 cases and corneal abscess in 1 case. The diagnosis of Acanthamoeba keratitis was based on corneal scraping in 2 cases, histology in 2 cases, and clinical findings in 2 cases.

Treatment started with antiamoebic agents in all patients: dibromopropamide or propamidin and polihexamethilen biguanidine was administered hourly in the first week, and then 5 times/day for at least 6 months. All patients were administered antibiotic drops 5 times a day for 2 weeks. We used steroid or non-steroid agents against the inflammation in seven cases.

In one case we performed corneal abrasion, but as it proved ineffective we followed it up with perforating keratoplasty.

Altogether penetrating keratoplasty was performed in six cases. In four cases keratoplasty was performed as an emergency (because of descemetocele) to save the eyeball, in two cases the operations were scheduled for visual rehabilitation.

All keratoplasties were perforating (penetrating), and central. All surgical procedures were done by two experienced surgeons. All cases were performed under retrobulbar anaesthesia. The trephination was performed with modified Geuder trephines. Donor corneas were obtained from the Eye Bank of our department. Only grafts with an endothelial cell count above 2000 cells/mm^2 were used. Graft fixation was performed in all cases with running nylon 10/0 sutures. We have had no intraoperative complications.

At the last follow up visit the average visual acuity was 0.43. In 3 cases it was only light perception, but the other 3 patients had very good corrected visual acuity (0.7-1.0).

In the emergency cases the visual acuity was much worse (light perception in 3 cases and 0.9 in one case, respectively), then in the proposed cases (0.7 and 1.0). In 5 cases the cornea graft was clear, rejection and decompensation developed only in one case.

Emergency keratoplasty is often the only possible intervention to prevent complete and irreversible vision loss in some cases. The main indications for this urgent surgical procedure are corneal perforations or imminent perforations, maintaining the integrity of the eyeball. Performing penetrating keratoplasty before scleral or peripheral corneal extension can minimize the risk of recurrence and poor outcome. Clear graft survival is lower if penetrating keratoplasty was performed during the acute, inflamed period of the disease compared to much higher clear graft survival when penetrating keratoplasty was performed in a quiet state of the disease. Perforating keratoplasty for visual restoration after resolution of *Acanthamoeba* keratitis in quiet eyes that are judged cyst-free by preoperative confocal microscopy appears to have an excellent long-term prognosis. Waiting at least 3 months after the discontinuation of medical therapy also appears helpful to rule out latent infection because of cyst reactivation and to allow the active inflammation to cease.

Acanthamoeba keratitis is a potentially blinding condition of the eye, and any steps toward prevention of this disease are encouraged. For prevention contact lens wearers are recommended to use daily disposable contact lenses to eliminate the contact lens case as a reservoir for Acanthamoeba. Hydrogen peroxide cleaning solutions are preferred over the more common multipurpose solutions. Planned replacement of contact lens storage cases may also help to reduce contamination. The rub and rinse step should be mentioned as the critical part of the disinfection. Detailed education of contact lens wearers concerning the entire disinfection procedure could minimize the incidence of Acanthamoeba keratitis further on. All of the eye care practitioners have to call attention of all contact lens users to aware the wearing of soft contact lenses in case of swimming so as to diminish the number of patients with Acanthamoeba keratitis. If even a soft contact lens wearer wants to swim, then daily disposable contact lens and swimming spectacles should be applied.

5. References

Amoils SP. & Heney C. (1999) Acanthamoeba keratitis with live isolates treatet with cryosurgery and Fluconazole. *Am. J. Ophthalmol*, Vol. 127, No. 6, pp. 718-720

Awwad ST., Parmar DN., Heilman M., Bowman RW., McCulley JP.& Cavanagh HD. (2005) Results of penetrating keratoplasty for visual rehabilitation after acanthamoeba keratitis. *Am J Ophthalmol*, Vol. 140, No. 6, pp. 1080-1084

Bacon AS., Frazer DG., Dart JKG., Mathelson M., Ficker LA. &Wright P.(1993) A review of 72 consecutive cases of Acanthamoeba keratitis. 1984-1992. *Eye*, Vol. 7, pp. 719-725

Beattie TK., Tomlinson A., & Mc Fadyen AK. (2006) Attachment of Acanthamoeba to first- and second-generation silicone hydrogel contact lenses. *Ophthalmology*, Vol. 113, No. 1, pp. 117-125

Beattie TK., Tomlinson A., McFadyen AK. Seal DV. & Grimason AM. (2003) Enhanced attachment of Acanthamoeba to extended-wear silicone hydrogel contact lenses. *Ophthalmology*, Vol. 110, No. 4, pp. 765-771

Bourcier T., Patteau F., Borderie V., Baudrimont M., Rondeau N., Bonnel S., Chaumeil C.& Laroche L. (2004) Amniotic membrane transplantation for the treatment severe acanthamoeba keratitis. *Can J Ophthalmol*, Vol. 39, No. 6, pp. 621-631

Chynn EW., Lopez MA., Pavan-Langston D. & Talamo JH. (1995) Acanthamoeba keratitis Contact lens and noncontact lens characteristic. *Ophthalmology*, Vol. 102, No.9, pp. 1369-1373

Clarke DW. & Niederkorn J. (2006) The pathophysiology of Acanthamoeba keratitis. *Trends Parasitol*, Vol. 22, No. 4, pp. 175-180

Cremona G., Carrasco MA., Tytiun A.&Cosentino MJ. (2002) Treatment of advanced Acanthamoeba keratitis with deep lamellar keratectomy and conjunctival flap. *Cornea*, Vol. 21, No. 7, pp. 705-708

Dart JK., Saw VP., & Kilvington S. (2009) Acanthamoeba keratitis: diagnosis and treatment update 2009. *Am J Ophthalmol*, Vol. 148, No. 4 pp. 487-499

Dejaco-Ruhswurm I., Scholz U., Hanselmayer G. & Skorpik C. (2001) Contact lens induced keratitis associated with contact lens wear. *Acta Ophthalmol Scand*, Vol. 79, pp. 479-483

Dunand VA., Hammer SM., Rossi R., Poulin M., Albrecht MA., Doweiko JP., DeGirolami PC., Coakley E., Piessens E. & Wanke CA. (1997) Parasitic sinusitis and otitis in patients infected with human immunodeficiency virus: report of five cases and review. *Clin Infect Dis*, Vol. 25, pp. 267-272

Ficker LA., Kirkness C.& Wright P. (1993) Prognosis for keratoplasty in Acanthamoeba keratitis. *Ophthalmology*, Vol. 100, No. 1, pp. 105-110

Gordon VR., Asem EK., Vodkin MH., & McLaughlin GL. (1993) Acanthamoeba binds to extracellular matrix proteins in vitro. *Invest Ophthalmol Vis Sci*, Vol. 34, pp. 658–662

Gray TB., Curson R.M., Sherwarn JF.Rose PR. (1995) Acanthamoeba, bacterial, and fungal contamination of contact lens storage cases. *Br J Ophthalmol*, Vol 79, pp. 601-605

Gullett J., Mills J., Hadley K., Podemski B., Pitts L. & Gelber R. (1979) Disseminated granulomatosus Acanthamoeba infection presenting as an unusual skin lesion. *Am J Med*, Vol. 67 pp. 891-896

Hahn TW., O'Brien TP., Sah WJ.& Kim JH. (1998) Acridine orange staining for rapid diagnosis of Acanthamoeba keratitis. *Jpn J Ophthalmol*, Vol. 42, No. 2, pp. 108-114

Hurt M., Niederkorn J., & Alizadeh H. (2003) Effects of mannose on Acanthamoeba castellanii proliferation and cytolytic ability to corneal epithelial cells. *Invest Ophthalmol Vis Sci*, Vol. 44, No. 8, pp. 3424-3431

Illingworth CD. & Cook SD. (1998) Acanthamoeba keratitis. *Surv Ophthalmol*, Vol. 42, No.6, pp. 493-508

Illingworth CD., Cook SD., Karabatsas CH. & Easty DL. (1995) Acanthamoeba keratitis risk factor and outcome. *Br J Ophthalmol*, Vol. 79, pp. 1078-1082

Jones BR., Visvesvara GS., & Robinson NM. (1975) Acanthamoeba polyphaga keratitis and Acanthamoeba uveitis associated with fatal meningoencephalitis. *Trans Ophthalmol Soc UK*, Vol. 95, pp. 221-232

Kaji Y., Hu B., Kawana K., & Oshika T. (2005) Swimming with soft contact lenses: danger of acanthamoeba keratitis. *Lancet Infect Dis*.Vol.5, No. 6, pp.392

Kashiwabuchi RT., de Freitas D., Alvarenga LS., Vieira L., Contarini P., Sato E., Foronda A. & Hofling-Lima AL. (2008) Corneal graft survival after therapeutic keratoplasty for Acanthamoeba keratitis. *Acta Ophthalmol*, Vol.86, No. 6, pp. 666-669

Kettesy B., Módis L., Komár T., Berta A. (2010) Acanthamoeba keratitis in patients with contact lens wear in the Department of Ophthalmology in Debrecen]. *Ophthalmologe*. Vol. 107, No. 6 pp.537-542

Khan NA. (2001) Pathogenicity, morphology, and differentation of Acanthamoeba. *Curr Microbiol*, Vol. 43, No. 6, pp. 391-395

Khan NA., Jarroll EL. & Paget TA. (2001) Acanthamoeba can be differentiated by the polymerase chain reaction and simple planting assay. *Curr Microbiol*, Vol. 43, No. 3, pp. 204-208

Kilvington S. (1993) Acanthamoeba trophozoite and cyst adherence to four types of soft contact lens and removal by cleaning agents. *Eye*, Vol. 7, pp. 535-538

Kilvington S., Gray T., Dart J., Moret N., Beechiing JR., Frazer DG. & Matheson M. (2004) Acanthamoeba keratitis: The role of domestic tap water contamination in the United Kingdom. *Invest Ophthalmol Vis Sci*, Vol. 45, No. 1, pp. 165-169

Kim JS., Kim JC., Na BK.,Jeong JM. &Song CY. (2000) Amniotic membrane patching promotes healing and inhibits proteinase activity on wound healing following acute corneal alkali burn. *Exp Eye Res*, Vol, 70, pp. 329-337

Kitzmann AS., Goins KM., Sutphin JE.& Wagoner MD. (2009) Keratoplasty for treatment of Acanthamoeba keratitis. *Ophthalmology*, Vol.116, No. 5, pp. 864-869

Lema I., Rodríguez-Ares MT., Gómez-Torreiro M. & Penalver MD. (2001) Adherence of Acanthamoeba to unworn conventional and disposable soft contact lenses. *Cornea,* Vol. 20, No. 6, pp. 635-638

Maier P., Böhringer D.& Reinhard T. (2007) Clear graft survival and immune reactions following emergency keratoplasty. *Graefes Arch Clin Exp Ophthalmol,* Vol. 245, No. 3, pp.351-359

Marciano-Cabral F., & Cabral G. (2003) Acanthamoeba ssp. as agent of disease in humans. *Clin Microbiol Rev,* Vol. 16, No. 2, pp. 273-307

Martinez AJ., Guerra AE., Garcia-Tamayo J., Céspedes G., Gonzalez-Alfonzo JE.&Visvesvara GS. (1994) Granulomatosus amoebic encephalitis: a review and report of a spontaneous case from Venezuela. *Acta Neuropathol,* Vol 87, No.4, pp. 430-434

Mc-Clellan K., Howard K., Niederkorn JY., & Alizadeh H. (2001) Effect of seroid on Acanthamoeba cyst and trophosoites. *Invest Ophthalmol Vis Sci,* Vol. 42, No. 12 pp. 2885-2893

Nagington J., Watson PG., Playfair TJ., McGill J., Jones BR. & Steele AD. (1974) Amoebic infection of the eye. *Lancet,* pp. 1537-1540

Nguyen TH., Weisenthal RW., Florakis GJ., Reidy JJ.,Gaster RN., & Tom D. (2010) Penetrating Keratoplasty in Active Acanthamoeba Keratitis. *Cornea,* Vol. 29, No. 9, pp. 1000-1004

Nwachuku N. & Gerba CP (2004) Health Effects of Acanthamoeba spp. and its potential for waterborne transmission. *Rev Environ Contam Toxicol,* Vol. 180, pp. 93-131

Parthasarathy A. & Tan DT. (2007) Deep lamellar keratoplasty for acanthamoeba keratitis. *Cornea,* Vol. 26, No. 8, pp. 1021-1023

Por YM., Mehta JS., Chua JL., Koh TH., Khor WB., Fong AC., Lim JW., Heng WJ., Loh RS., Lim L. & Tan DT. (2009) Acanthamoeba keratitis associated with contact lens wear in Singapore. *Am J Ophthalmol,* Vol. 148, No. 1, pp. 7-12

Qian Y., Meisler DM., Langston RH.& Jeng BH. (2010) Clinical experience with Acanthamoeba keratitis at the cole eye institute, 1999-2008. *Cornea,* Vol. 29, No. 9, pp. 1016-1021

Radford CF., Bacon AS., Dart JKG., & Minassian DC. (1995) Risk factors for acanthamoeba keratitis contact lens users: a case control study. *BMJ,* Vol. 310 pp.1567–1570

Radford CF., Lehmann OJ., & Dart JKG. (1998) Acanthamoeba keratitis: multicentre survey in England 1992–1996. *Br J Ophthalmol,* Vol. 82j pp.1387–1392

Radford CF., Minassian DC., & Dart JKG. (2002) Acanthamoeba keratitis in England and Wales: incidence, outcome, and risk factors. *Br J Ophthalmol,* Vol. 86j pp. 536–542

Reinhard T., & Sundmacher R. (2000) Klinik und Therapie der Akantamöbenkeratitis. *Ophthalmologe,* Vol. 97, pp. 446-459

Seal DV. 2003 Acanthamoeba keratitis update-incidence, molecular epidemiology and new drugs for treatment. *Eye,* Vol.17, pp. 893-905

Seal DV., Kirkness CM., Bennett HGB. & Peterson M. (1999) Acanthamoeba keratitis in Scotland: risk factors for contact lens wearers. *Contact Lens Anterior Eye,* Vol. 22, No. 2, pp. 58-68

Sharma S., Garg P. & Rao GN. (2000) Patient characteristics, diagnosis, and treatment of non-contact lens releated Acanthamoeba keratitis. *Br J Ophthalmol,* Vol. 84, pp. 1103-1108

Shi W., Liu M., Gao H., Li S. & Xie L. (2009) Perioperative treatment and prognostic factors for penetrating keratoplasty in Acanthamoeba keratitis unresponsive to medical treatment. *Graefes Arch Clin Exp Ophthalmol*, Vol. 247, No. 10, pp. 1383-1388

Shih KL., Hu J.& Sibley MJ. (1985) The microbiological benefit of cleaning and rinsing of contact lenses. *Int Contact Lens Clin*; Vol. 12. pp.235–242.

Stehr-Green JK., Bailey TM., & Visvesvara GS. (1989) The epidemiology of Acanthamoeba keratitis in the United States. *Am J Ophthalmol*, Vol. 107, No. 4, pp. 331–336

Taenaka N, Fukuda M, Hibino T, Kato Y, Arimura E, Ishii Y, & Shimomura Y. (2007) Surgical therapies for Acanthamoeba keratitis by phototherapeutic keratectomy and deep lamellar keratoplasty. *Cornea*, Vol. 26, No. 7, pp. 876-879

Tanhehco T.& Colby K. (2010) The clinical experience of Acanthamoeba keratitis at a tertiary care eye hospital. *Cornea*,Vol.29, No.9, pp.1005-1010

Wilhelmus KR., Jones DB., Matoba AY., Hamill MB., Pflugfelder SC., & Weikert MP.Bilateral acanthamoeba keratitis. *Am J Ophthalmol*, 2008 Vol. 145, No. 2, pp. 193-197

Part 2

Lamellar Keratoplasties

4

Manual Deep Anterior Lamellar Keratoplasty

Farid Daneshgar
Kermanshah University of Medical Sciences
Iran

1. Introduction

Keratoplasty is considered the most successful organ transplantation procedure in the world. Reisinger was the first to use the term keratoplasty (Reisinger, 1824), when he suggested using an animal's eye to provide donor corneal tissue for corneal transplantation in a human. In 1906, the first successful penetrating keratoplasty was performed by Edward Konrad Zirm on a patient suffering from bilateral alkali burns (Zirm, 1906). Ramon Castroviego created some fine instruments that were named after him and was the first to perform successful penetrating keratoplasty using fine sutures (Castroviejo, 1932). His square-shaped grafts survived for many years and provided good vision for his patients.

In 1886, Von Hipple erformed lamellar corneal transplantation (Von Hipple, 1888). The concept of deep lamellar corneal dissection and leaving the Descemet membrane (DM) intact was first proposed by Von Walther and was described further by Muhlbauer (Muhlbauer, 1824). A full-thickness donor corneal tissue without any dissection through the corneal stromal tissue was proposed for lamellar keratoplasty in 1959 (Hallermann, 1963). Hallermann proposed both full-thickness donor graft with the endothelium (FTDGE) and full-thickness donor graft without the endothelium (FTDG) over a deeply dissected corneal stromal recipient's bed for lamellar keratoplasty. Morrison and Swan provided histopathologic evidence that FTDG is associated with less inflammation and scarring than FTDGE (Morrison & Swan, 1982).

Today, removing the corneal stromal tissues down to the DM or the pre-Descemet membrane level and using a FTDG is the standard of care for patients requiring deep anterior lamellar keratoplasty (DALK) surgery. Many techniques have been developed for performing DALK surgery. Before reviewing some surgical techniques for the procedure, I will discuss some factors that influence the visual outcomes.

2. Major factors influencing the visual outcome after DALK surgery

2.1 Clear donor tissue

The purpose of lamellar corneal transplantation is to substitute the diseased parts of the cornea by a clear donor tissue.

2.2 Clear remaining corneal tissue in recipient

A corneal surgeon must be vigilant to remove every opacified or scar tissue from the stromal bed. Involvement of the DM and adjacent tissues with scarring could be considered a contraindication for DALK surgery.

2.3 Deep plane of recipient's corneal stromal dissection

Lamellar corneal grafts are classified according to the depth of dissection through the recipient's corneal stromal tissues.

2.3.1 Superficial anterior lamellar keratoplasty (SALK)

The dissection plane is up to 160 μm or about 30% of corneal thickness from the surface.

2.3.2 Mid-anterior lamellar keratoplasty (MALK)

The dissection plane is from 160 to 400 μm or about 30% to 70% of corneal thickness from the surface.

2.3.3 Deep anterior lamellar keratoplasty (DALK)

The dissection plane is 400 μm from the surface to the DM. However, from the terminology viewpoint, the term maximum-depth anterior lamellar keratoplasty (MD-ALK) is used when the bare DM is exposed in the recipient's cornea and the term total anterior lamellar keratoplasty (TALK) is used when the bare DM is exposed in the recipient's entire corneal bed and no remaining corneal stromal tissue is present within the trephination wound area.

Generally, the wound repair process is accompanied by more scar formation and opacification in the superficial corneal stromal layers compared to the deep corneal stromal layers. So the deeper the dissection plane in the recipient's corneal stromal tissues, the lower is the risk of irregularities and scarring in the interface.

2.4 Smooth posterior surface of donor tissue

The smoothest posterior surface of the donor tissue is provided when no dissection cuts through the stromal tissues, FTDG is used, and the DM and endothelial cells are wiped out gently.

2.5 Smooth anterior surface of recipient's tissue

The smoothest surface of recipient's bed is provided when the bare DM is exposed in the recipient's cornea.

2.6 Clear interface

The interface between donor and recipient tissues should be washed thoroughly to eliminate the risk of any retained material in the interface, such as viscoelastic material or filaments especially over the optical zone of the cornea.

2.7 Uniform thickness of donor tissue throughout the graft area

Because the normal corneal thickness gradually increases from the central area toward the peripheral area, great care must be taken to avoid any decentration of the donor tissue when it is cut by a corneal punch. Decentered punching of the donor cornea will result in a donor button that has different thicknesses around the edge of its circumference.

2.8 Uniform thickness of recipient's tissue throughout the graft area

Many corneal surgeons focus their attention on removing the corneal stromal tissues over the central area to expose the bare DM. They may pay little attention to removing adequate stromal tissues near the trephination wound to make a uniform thickness recipient bed for transplantation. It should be emphasized that removing adequate stromal tissues near the trephination wound is as important, if not more important, than doing so in the central cornea. If the task is not performed, the Bowman-to-Bowman opposition of the donor and recipient will occur by excessive force over the sutures and unpredictable visual results will occur when sutures are removed or when sutures lose their tensile strength. The ideal situation is provided by the TALK procedure in which the DM is exposed in the entire trephination wound area. In TALK cases, early removal of corneal sutures can be accompanied with good visual results.

2.9 Minimal irregularities of the anterior surface of the donor tissue over the optical zone

Given a donor cornea devoid of any preexisting pathology, the corneal sutures will be the major source of irregularities of the anterior corneal surface. In fact, the irregularities originate from the suture sites and radiate over the corneal surface vanishing toward the central area. So the further the distance between a given point over the corneal surface and a suture site, the less the amount of irregularity at the specific point.

If we liken the irregularities that originate from the sutures to the cold winds and the optical zone to a freezing man, it could be said that cold wind of irregularities blow from the suture sites toward the optical zone so the best way to protect the freezing man in the optical zone from the cold wind of irregularities will be to put it at the center of the circle (Figure 1)

Hence, selection of the pupil center as the center of the trephination wound protects the optical zone from adverse effects of the sutures all around the wound.

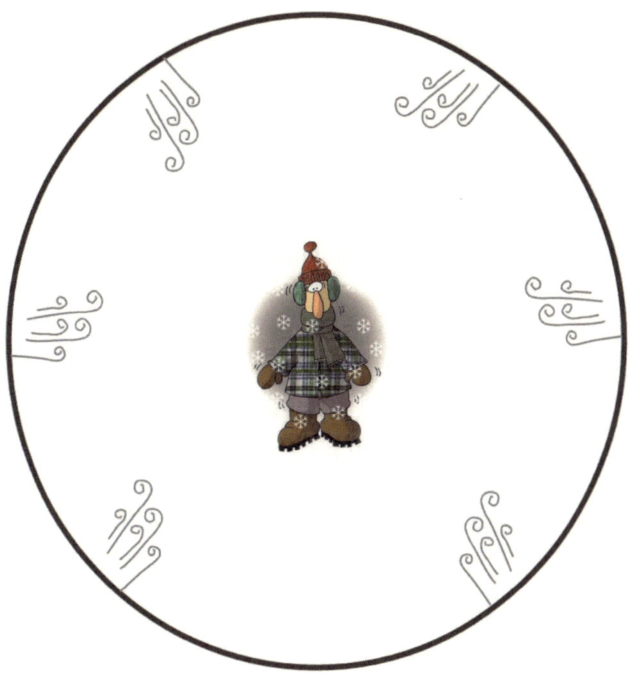

Fig. 1. Visual axis can be kept away from the sutures at the center of the circle just as the Freezing man keep himself away from the cold winds.

3. Indications for optical DALK surgery

DALK is indicated for conditions associated with opacification of the corneal stromal tissues over the central area of the cornea while the DM and endothelium are normal and not involved. The opacification may be due to trauma, infections, iatrogenic causes, chemical insults, dystrophies, or degenerations.
DALK is also used for ectatic corneal disorders with normal DM and endothelium, such as keratoconus, keratoglobus, pellucid marginal degeneration, or ectasia occurring after LASIK surgery.

4. Surgical techniques

The superiorities of DALK over penetrating keratoplasty cannot be overemphasized. However, for obtaining best results, a corneal surgeon must be familiar with different surgical maneuvers used for performing DALK. In this overview of some techniques for performing DALK, some surgical "pearls" will enrich our repertoire of skills.

4.1 Using air to perform DALK

In 1984, Arenas introduced the concept of injecting air into the corneal stroma for performing DALK and the technique was named air-deep lamellar keratoplasty (AD-LKP) (Arenas, 1985). He injected air into superficial corneal stromal tissues at the peripheral cornea. Then a partial-thickness trephination cut of about 400 μm was performed in the resultant emphysematous, white corneal tissue. The superficial corneal layers were removed using sharp blades and deep stromal layers were removed using blunt spatulas until reaching the pre-Descemet level. The movement of the spatulas was centripetally starting at the wound margins and ending at the center or thinnest part of the cornea. He described the pre-Descemet layer as a black and shiny surface devoid of air. The DM was not exposed by this technique; however, after long-term follow-up, the visual results were better than those for penetrating keratoplasty.

4.2 Using shearing and traction force instead of cutting to perform DALK

Malbran introduced the peeling-off technique (Malbran, 1966). His concept of a peeling rather than a cutting action for removing the recipient's corneal stromal tissues provided a smoother surface that served as the bed for transplantation. In this technique, the stromal tissues are pooled in a direction that is perpendicular to the corneal surface and a semi-sharp instrument leads the direction of shearing of tissue through the corneal stromal layers. He also modified his technique by combining it with intrastromal air injection. The intrastromal air facilitates tissue removal and also provides some assistance for differentiating the pre-Descemet layer from more superficial stromal layers. He used the pre-Descemet layer as the bed for the FTDG while he did the DALK procedure. He performed large-diameter grafts (9-10 mm) and reported that the astigmatism was usually regular from the first postoperative day. It seems that large-diameter grafts provide enough distance between suture sites and the visual axis to protect it from cold winds of irregularity (Factor 9 above). In my experience, regular astigmatism on the first postoperative day can be obtained with an 8-mm wound area if the center of the trephination wound has been set over the pupil center.

4.3 Using fluid to perform DALK

Sugita and Kondo introduced the technique of hydrodelamination (Sugita & Kondo, 1997). They injected a balanced salt solution (BSS) into the stromal bed after a lamellar dissection of the cornea. The injection made the stromal collagen fibers swell. A spatula was introduced into the hydrated area and the stroma was dissected by moving the spatula in a fanlike motion. They called this maneuver "spatula delamination." The overlying dissected tissues were removed and the maneuver was repeated until the bare DM was reached in the central cornea. This technique has the advantage of discriminating between normal and pathologic cornea because the pathologic cornea (usually scar) does not swell as well as the normal cornea when being hydrated. This allows the surgeon to determine the depth of the pathology in the corneal stroma.

4.4 Using air and fluid to perform DALK

Anwar and Teichmann combined the use of air and fluid for planned near-Descemet membrane dissection for performing DALK (Anwar & Teichmann, 2002). They recommended that this technique be used in patients in whom exposing the DM carries a high risk of DM perforation. Such conditions include deep corneal scars involving the DM, patients with keratoconus who have experienced hydrops, those with known DM fragility such as macular dystrophy, and inexperienced corneal surgeons performing occasional lamellar grafts. They created some swelling in the stromal bed after a lamellar dissection by hydrating the stromal collagen fibers. They injected air into the swollen area and removed the resultant emphysematous tissues using Anwar's keratoplasty spatula and repeated the maneuver until they reached the pre-Descemet layer. They described the layer as a semitransparent tissue with the pupil and iris pattern visible through the layer. They concluded that the risk of DM rupture is lower with this technique compared to injecting air alone because the hydrated tissues are thickened and introducing the needle and spatula into the thickened tissue carries a lower risk of violating the DM.

4.5 Using viscoelastic material for performing DALK

Manche and colleagues used viscoelastic material for separating the DM from the overlying stromal tissues (Manche et al., 1999). They used forceful injection of the viscoelastic material into a pocket incision to make a cleavage plane between the DM and posterior stroma. The pocket was made by a Paufique knife and was parallel to the stromal collagen fibers. Melles and coworkers described the "air-to-endothelium" light reflex as a guide for approaching the DM—stroma interface (Melles et al., 1999). They described a "dark band" between the blade tip and a specular light reflex as the non-incised stromal tissue before reaching the DM—stroma interface. By advancing the blade tip through the dark band the custom-made blade reached the DM—stroma interface and they redirected the blade parallel to the interface to separate the overlying tissues. In 2002, Melles and colleagues introduced the visco-dissection DALK (Melles et al., 2002). They injected viscoelastic material directly over the DM using the air-to-endothelium light reflex as a guide for precise location of the injection for making a DM detachment over an area that was going to be cut by a vacuum trephine. In fact, a TALK procedure has been performed by removing the overlying tissues and using the FTDG.

4.6 Using dye for performing DALK

Balestrazzi and colleagues used a 0.02% solution of trypan blue for staining the stromal collagen fibers (Balestrazzi et al., 2002). This facilitated the discrimination of the stromal fibers from underlying DM. John used indocyanine green and forced hydrodissection for performing TALK (John, 2004). This technique benefits from both hydrating the collagen fibers to create stromal swelling for introducing spatulas into the stromal tissues safely and using dye for discriminating the stromal fibers from the underlying DM.

4.7 Using air for DM detachment in performing DALK

Anwar and Teichmann introduced the big-bubble technique for performing DALK (Anwar & Teichmann, 2002). The technique is a fast method for separating the DM from corneal stroma. The air is injected in the deep layers of the corneal stromal tissues after a partial-thickness trephination cut of about 60% to 80% of the corneal thickness. In most cases a big bubble is formed at the DM—stroma interface and a circular white outline demarcates the borders of the air bubble. The overlying corneal tissues are removed to expose the DM and provide the recipient bed for performing MD-ALK. This technique is used by many corneal surgeons throughout the world for performing DALK.

Large-bubble modified technique for performing DALK was introduced in 2010 (Behrooz & Daneshgar, 2010). The rationale of this technique was to create an air bubble at the DM—stroma interface that was larger than the trephination wound so that total removal of the corneal stromal tissues could be accomplished with scissors to perform the TALK procedure. The "expanding-bubble modification of the big-bubble technique" (Daneshgar & Fallahtafti, 2011) is the method that I believe is useful for providing full exposure of the DM and performing TALK. The procedure is performed as follows:

A partial-thickness trephination to a depth of about 60% to 80% of the corneal thickness is performed as described in the big-bubble technique (Anwar & Teichmann, 2002). The center of the pupil is determined as the center of trephination using an 8- to 8.25- calibrated trephine (Katena Products, Denville, NJ) for an average cornea (Figures 2 and 3).

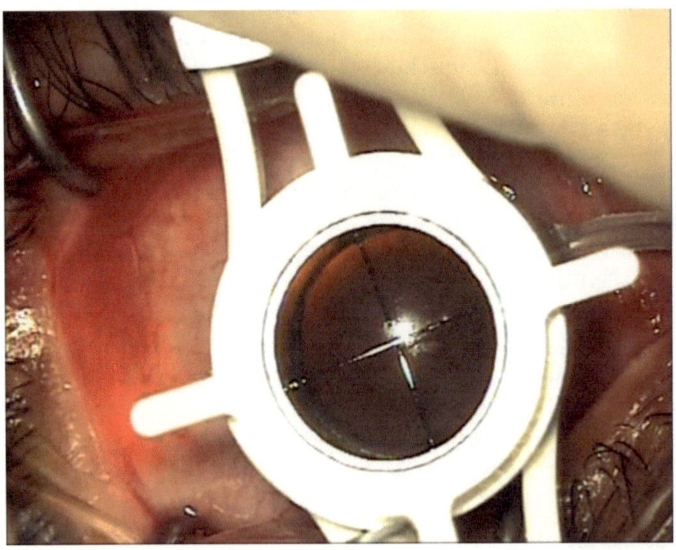

Fig. 2. Center of the pupil is considered as the center for trephination cut. Note that the pupil is dilated due to the injection of retrobulbar anesthetic solution.

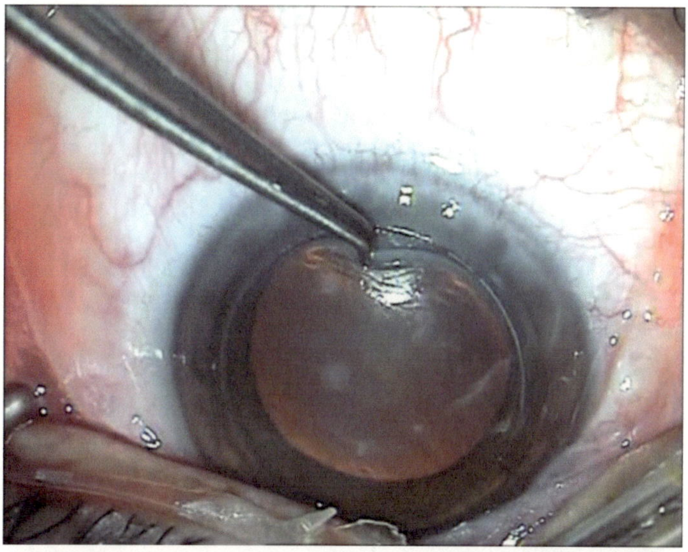

Fig. 3. Depth of the trephination wound is checked using a fine toothed forceps.

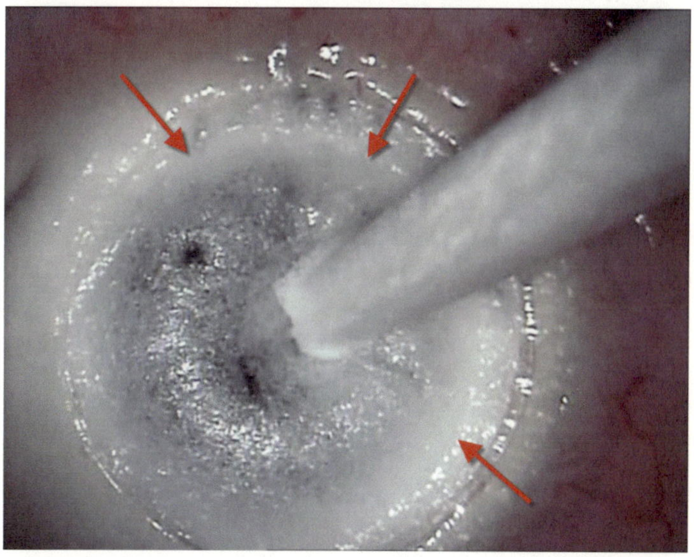

Fig. 4. Sunny side up sign, red arrows point at a circular furrow encircling the air bubble at the DM_ stroma interface.

A 27-gauge needle attached to an air-filled syringe is inserted bevel down into the deep stroma in the paracentral cornea as in the big-bubble technique. After air is injected, a paracentesis wound is performed using a stab knife (Eagle Laboratories, Rancho Cucamonga, CA) in a semivertical direction to drain aqueous fluid. A crescent blade (Eagle Laboratories) is used to excise emphysematous stromal tissues as in lamellar keratectomy. The paracentesis wound is widened to 3 mm with the stab knife and the posterior lip of the wound is depressed to drain some aqueous fluid to make the anterior chamber obviously hypotensive. A dry Weck-Cel® sponge is used to depress the cornea. When a big bubble

forms, the outline of the bubble is obviously seen as a circular furrow around a dome-shaped elevation in the center, similar to the yolk of a sunny-side up egg (Figure 4).
This sunny-side up sign is useful for determining the presence and extent of the air bubble. The diameter of the bubble can easily be measured using calipers. In most instances the diameter of the bubble is about 6 to 7 mm and the border of the air bubble coincides with the trephination wound inferiorly and lies within about 2 mm inside the trephination wound superiorly (Figure 4). It may also be smaller in size, usually when repeated attempts at air injection have been needed (Figure 5),
It may form eccentrically as the bubble border extends beyond the trephination wound over a specific area and lies within the trephination wound in some other area (Figure 6).

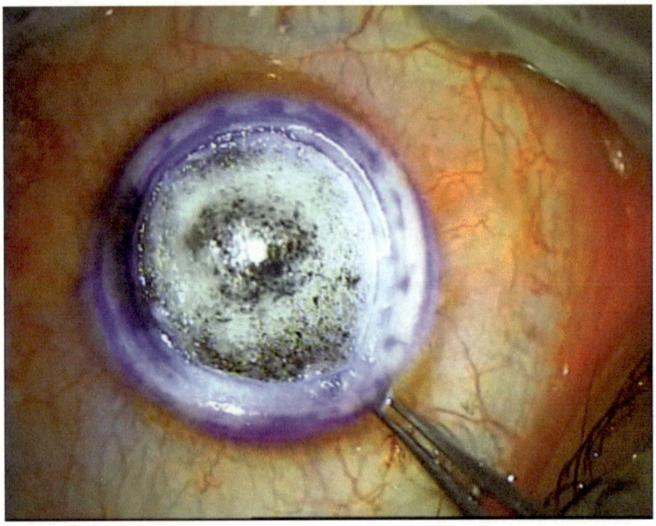

Fig. 5. Sunny side up sign with a small egg yoke.

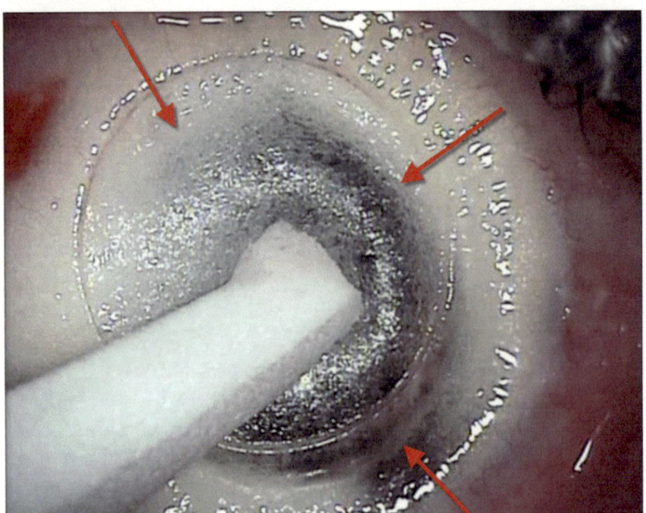

Fig. 6. Eccentric big-bubble. The air bubble extends beyond the trephination wound inferiorly. Red Arrows point at the boundries of the big-bubble.

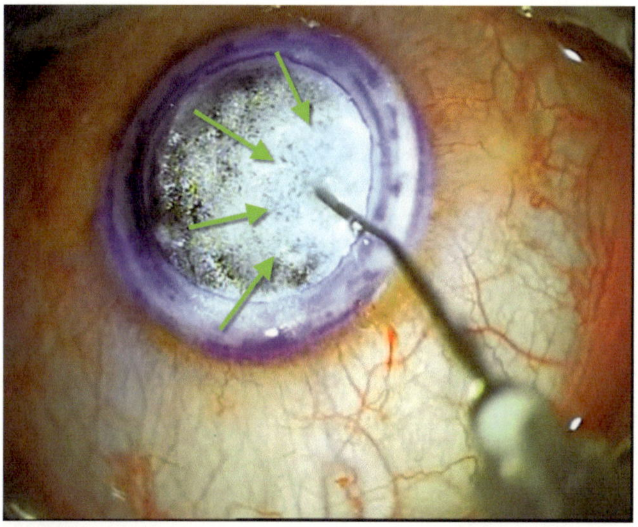

Fig. 7. Green arrows point at the hydrated area in the corneal stromal bed.

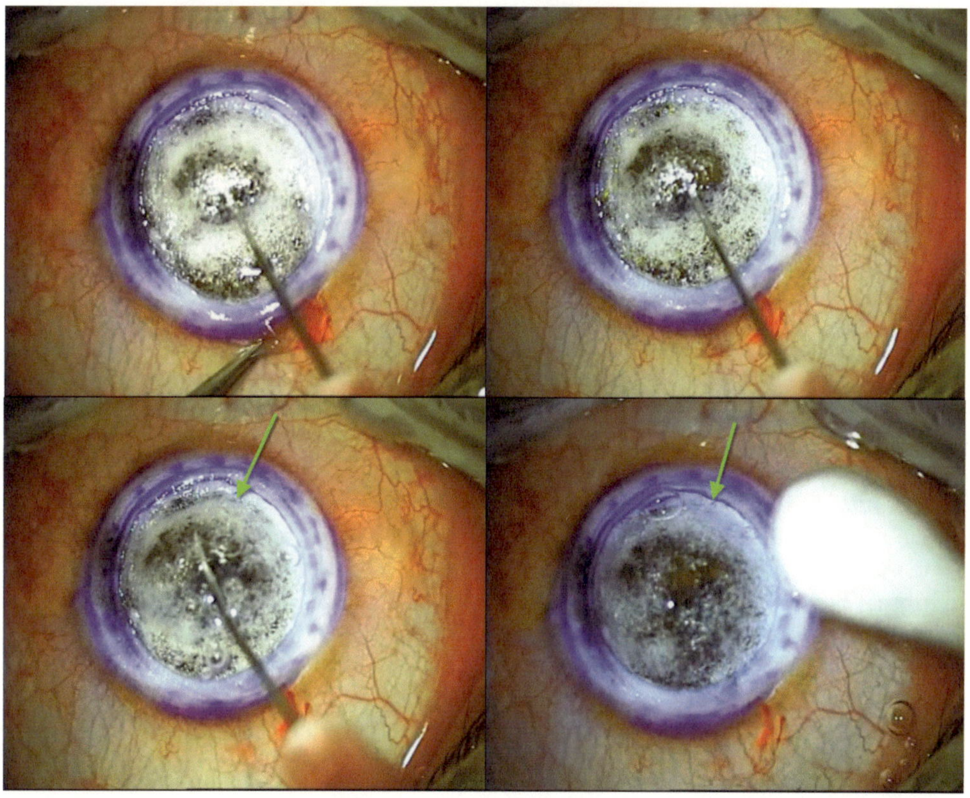

Fig. 8. The bubble is expanded by injecting viscoelastic material into the bubble cavity. Viscoelastic injection is discontinued and the needle is withdrawn when the demarcating furrow reaches the trephination wound circumference.

When no big bubble is formed, the procedure is continued by hydrating a localized area in the stroma with BSS. There is no need for introducing a needle into the corneal stromal tissues for hydrating the collagen fibers; instead we can use a blunt-tipped cannula attached to a syringe filled with BSS to hydrate the stromal tissues by putting the blunt tip in close contact with the stromal tissues in a perpendicular direction and injecting fluid while depressing the tissues by the tip of the cannula (Figure 7). Air injection is repeated in the hydrated area using the same 27-gauge needle and an air-filled syringe. After the sunny-side up sign is seen, the 27-gauge needle used for air injection is attached to a syringe containing viscoelastic material (Coatel™; Bausch & Lomb, Madison, NJ). Viscoelastic material is injected while the needle is inserted into the bubble cavity in the horizontal direction with a rapid movement.

The injection of the viscoelastic material into the bubble cavity is continued slowly as the "egg yolk" is expanded slowly (Figures 8-9).

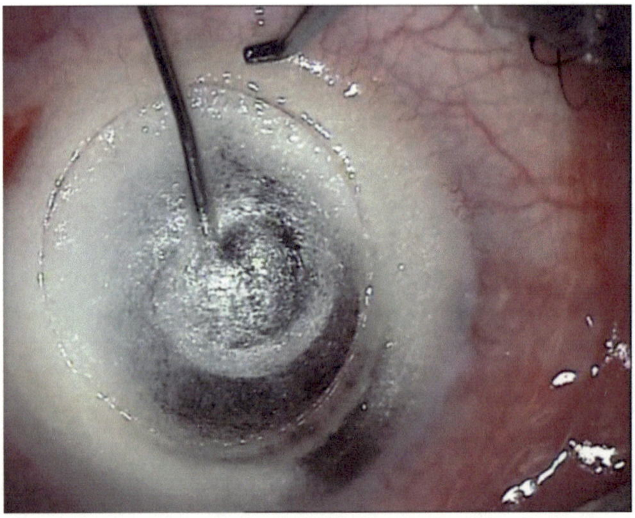

Fig. 9. Viscoelastic material is injected into the bubble cavity.

Care must be taken not to depress the cornea while injecting the viscoelastic material or to overexpand the bubble beyond the trephination wound because these actions may rupture the DM. Just as the demarcation furrow reaches the trephination wound margins, the injection of viscoelastic material is stopped and the needle is withdrawn. The stab knife is used to incise the roof of the bubble (Figure 10).

The stromal tissues at the anterior wall of the bubble are excised using curved blunt-tipped corneal scissors (18010; Moria, Antony, France) around the trephination wound circumference (Figure 11).

The DM is exposed to the full extent (Figure 12).

The donor tissue is prepared by disinserting the DM and endothelium from peripheral insertion using a dry Weck-Cel® sponge and wiping it off from the posterior surface of the corneal stroma. A vital dye can be used to stain the endothelium and DM for discriminating the layer from stromal tissues and easy removal of the layer, but I usually put the donor tissue over the back surface of a steel container. The shining reflex of the steel surface facilitates the visualization of the delicate DM (Figure 13).

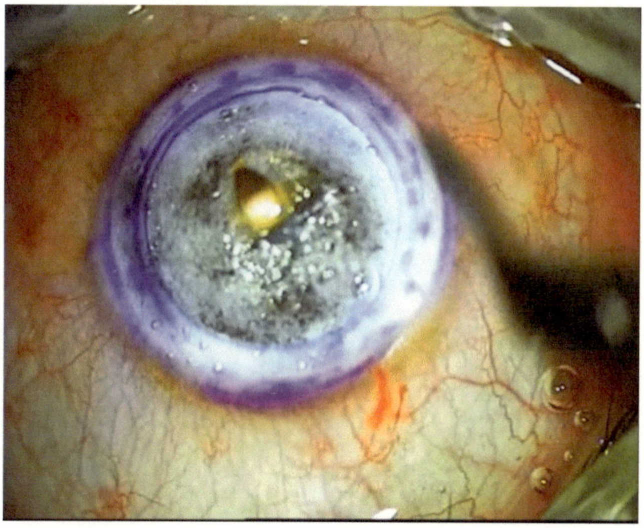

Fig. 10. Anterior wall of the bubble is incised using a stab knife.

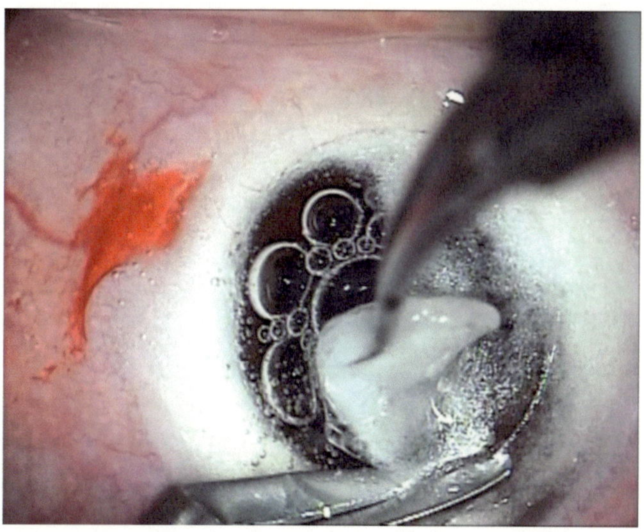

Fig. 11. Anterior wall of the bubble is excised using blunt tip curved scissors along the trephination wound circumference leaving no corneal stromal tissues within the trephination wound area.

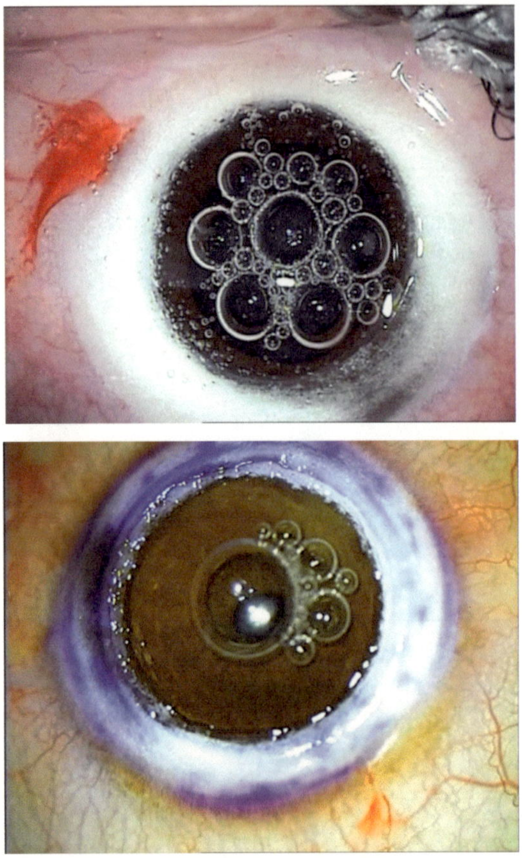

Fig. 12. Descemet mambrane is exposed troughout the entire trephination wound area.

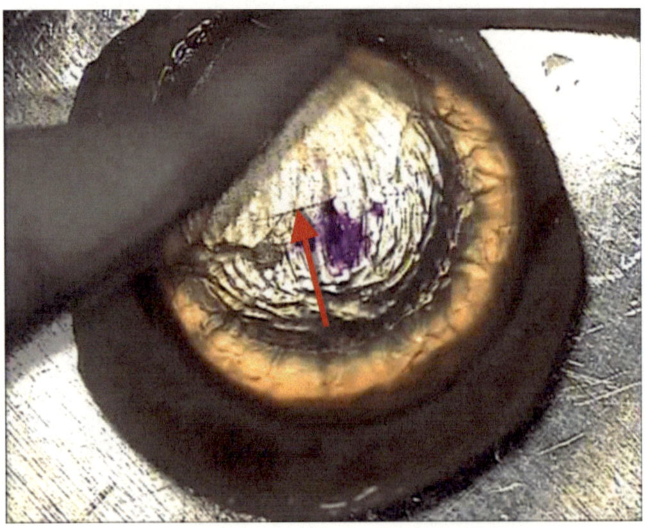

Fig. 13. Dry Weck-Cel sponge is used for disinserting DM from the peripheral insertions and wipping it off from posterior surface of the donor cornea.

After this stage no manipulation of the recipient's bed is allowed because no endothelium is present in the donor tissue for converting to penetrating keratoplasty if required. I always remove any residual episcleral and scleral tissues except a small rim around the limbus because those excessive tissues may cause decentered punching of the donor tissue if the punch is not equipped with a suction system (Figure 14).

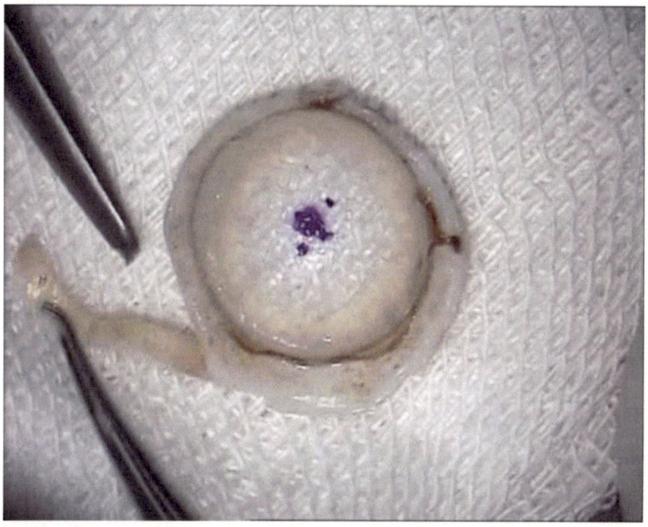

Fig. 14. Execcive scleral tissues are excised.

Conversely, care must be taken not to violate the limbus. Cutting the limbal tissues by scissors will result in an ellipsoid rather than round donor button. Loose corneal epithelium may result in donor tissue slippage and decentered punching if the donor tissue is not fresh.

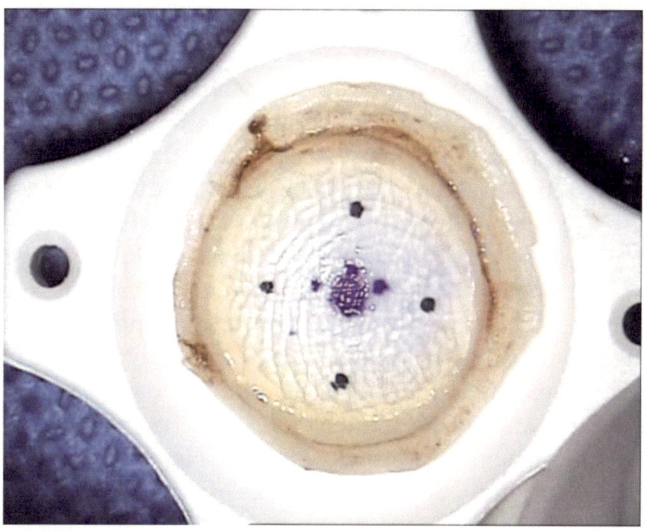

Fig. 15. Geometrical center of the donor cornea is considered as the center for cutting the donor tissue using a corneal punch.

Hence, if the corneal epithelium is loose and edematous it must be wiped away using an applicator. The precise geometric center of the donor cornea is determined and marked. The donor cornea devoid of endothelium is put in a corneal punch (Katena Products) using the mark for centration (Figure 15) and is cut to the desired size.

I routinely put some viscoelastic material over the punch blade before cutting, which is useful in creating a more even and smoother edge of the cut donor button. Conversely, the edge of the donor button might become "s" shaped especially if the punch blade is not sharp enough (Figure 16).

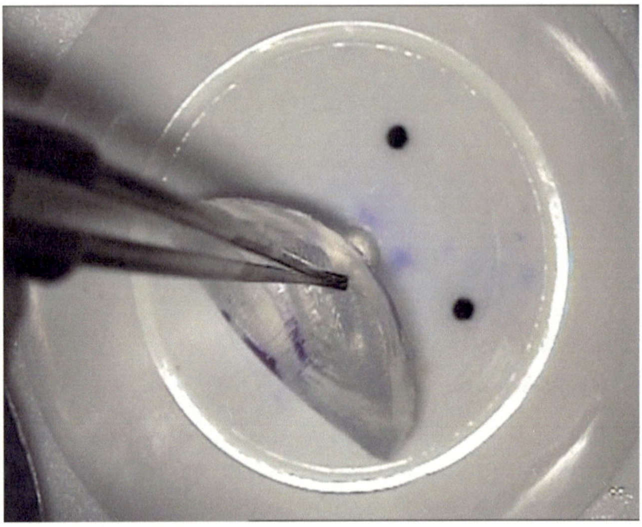

Fig. 16. A coin shape donor button with vertical edges is achieved.

Ultimately, the donor button is secured in the recipient site with sutures (10-0 nylon). The exposed surface of the DM is irrigated with free-flowing BSS for removing the viscoelastic material completely after placing the first corneal suture (Figure 17). I prefer to perform mixed continuous and separate sutures (Figures 18-20). In the TALK procedure the depth of the sutures traveling through the corneal tissues is identical at both sides of the graft interface and is approximately 80% to 90% of the corneal thickness at both donor and host tissue sides. If no big bubble is formed after several attempts at air injection, a deep lamellar dissection is performed with a crescent knife to the pre-Descemet level. The tiny air bubbles can be recognized at the DM—stroma interface under high microscopic magnification. The viscoelastic material is injected after inserting the tip of a 30-gauge needle attached to the viscoelastic syringe into a tiny bubble and the bubble will begin to expand. If the overlying collagen fibers are not removed sufficiently, the bubble will expand into the anterior chamber and the surgeon must drain the aqueous fluid from the anterior chamber to provide space for the bubble to expand. If the overlying collagen fibers are minimal, the bubble will expand over the DM toward the outer space and the procedure will continue as described above.

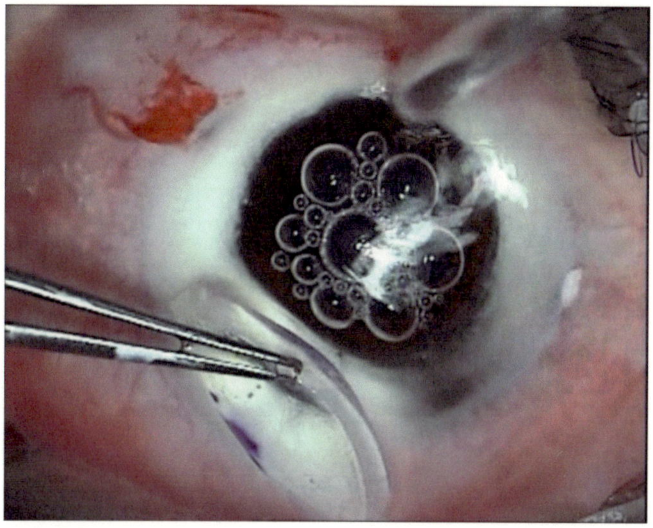

Fig. 17. The exposed surface of the DM is irrigated with free-flowing solution.

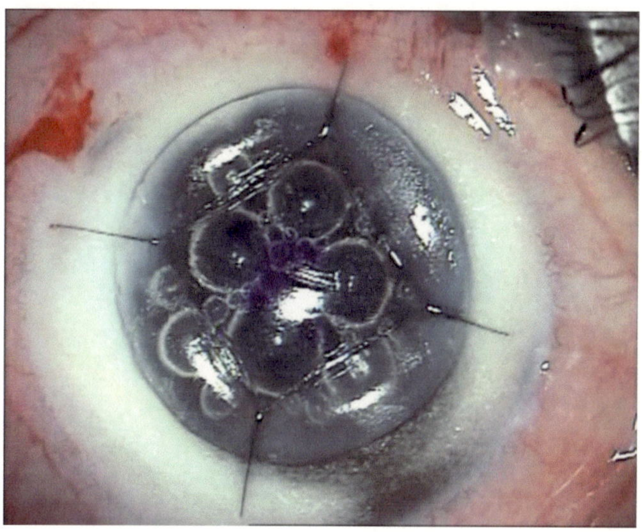

Fig. 18. Cardinal sutures are placed

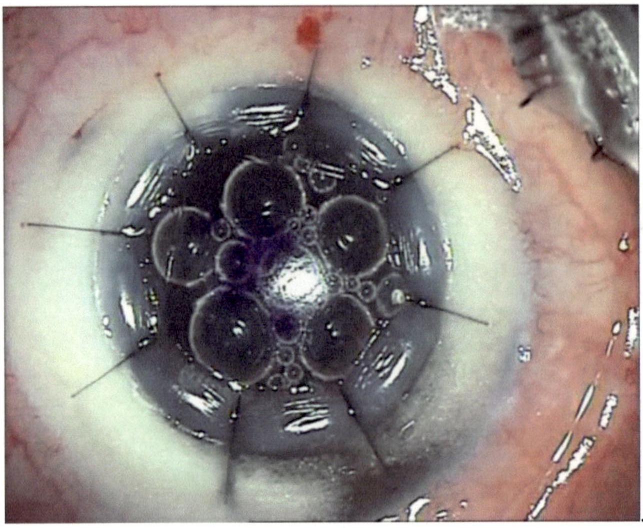

Fig. 19. Eight separate radial sutures are tied and Burried in the donor button.

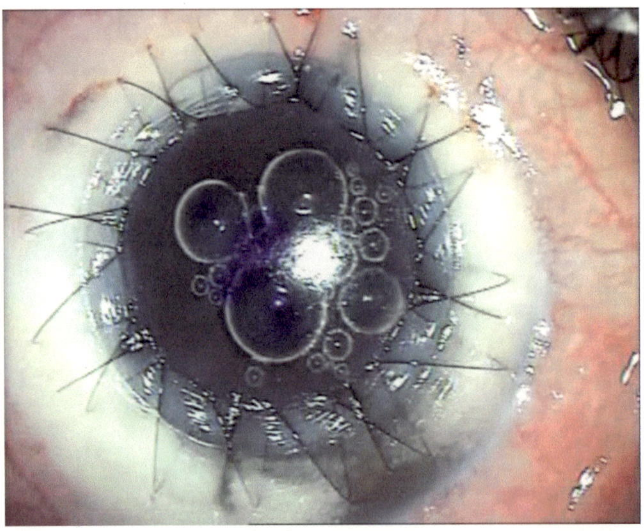

Fig. 20. Suturing the donor button in the recipient bed is completed using combined Interrupted and continuous sutures.

5. Follow-up schedule

The eye is examined on the first postoperative day and after a week. In these visits special attention is focused on the corneal epithelium. Usually a bandage soft lens and nonpreserved lubricant drops are used to improve reepithelialization of the cornea. Topical steroids and antibiotics are started on the first postoperative day. Topical antibiotics are discontinued after the epithelium heals completely. Topical steroids are tapered off over a 4-month period. The patient visits at monthly intervals for 4 months. During this period, every loose suture must be removed and replaced by a new suture. Adjustment of the tension of the continuous sutures can be performed during this period. After the fourth month the patient is examined every 2 months. At the 6-month postoperative visit and beyond the corneal sutures are selectively removed to improve visual function. I routinely remove sutures with the guide of retinoscopy alone and rarely a topographic corneal image is needed to determine the suture that requires removal. I remove the continuous suture if the spherical equivalent is over +3 and remove radial sutures along the steepest corneal meridian (the most "with movement" of the light reflex intercept while performing retinoscopy).

6. Complications

6.1 Perforation of the DM

Perforation of the DM can occur during trephination. In this instance the wound must be sutured and the operation is better postponed to a time after the wound has healed for planned pre-Descemet level DALK.

Perforation can also occur after penetration by the tip of the needle for air injection, in which case air immediately enters the anterior chamber. No attempt to expose the bare DM should be made. However, a pre-Descemet DALK could be performed in these cases.

When the large-bubble or expanding-bubble technique is used, perforation of the DM may occur after the DM—stroma interface is overfilled. A horizontal radial tear appears at the center of the DM along the 3-to-9 o'clock meridian. It is wise to convert these surgeries to penetrating keratoplasty because trying to oppose the DM to the posterior surface of the donor cornea using gas tamponade is difficult. Even if this procedure is successfully performed, it is associated with opacification and scar formation over an elliptical area (fish-mouth shape) in the posterior corneal surface that is devoid of DM. The opacification has adverse visual effects because it is centrally located.

Perforation of the DM can occur during lamellar dissection and tissue removal. In these cases a pre-Descemet DALK can be performed. The perforation site must be left until the end of tissue removal and a small amount of stromal tissue must be left over the perforation site to seal the perforation.

If an instrument touches the bare DM, perforation is possible. In most of these cases the procedure can be continued by thoroughly washing any retained viscoelastic material, suturing the donor tissue in place, and using air for intracameral injection to seal the perforation. Because the dome-shaped contour of the cornea is reduced, especially with tight sutures, the air bubble in the anterior chamber will apply noticeable pressure over the pupil to induce papillary block. Performing a peripheral iridotomy via a paracentesis is necessary and infusion of a hyperosmotic solution such as 20% mannitol is necessary to induce vitreous shrinkage if not contraindicated according to the patient's general status.

A small peripheral iridotomy will not guarantee that the patient will not experience a relative papillary block if the air bubble is so large or if expanding gas such as SF_6or C_3F_8 is used.

6.2 Double anterior chamber

Double anterior chamber occurs when a perforation is present in the recipient's bed. If the amount of fluid in the interface is minimal, the condition can be managed by observation alone. If not, the intracameral injection of air or gas (SF_6or C_3F_8) and the drainage of the interface fluid can manage the condition. Great care must be taken to not inject air over the DM in the interface. Every effort must be made to prevent papillary block.

6.3 Foreign particles within the interface

Foreign particles in the interface can be left in place without any attempt to remove them if there has been no associated inflammation and edema and they have been out of the optical zone of the cornea (Figure 21).

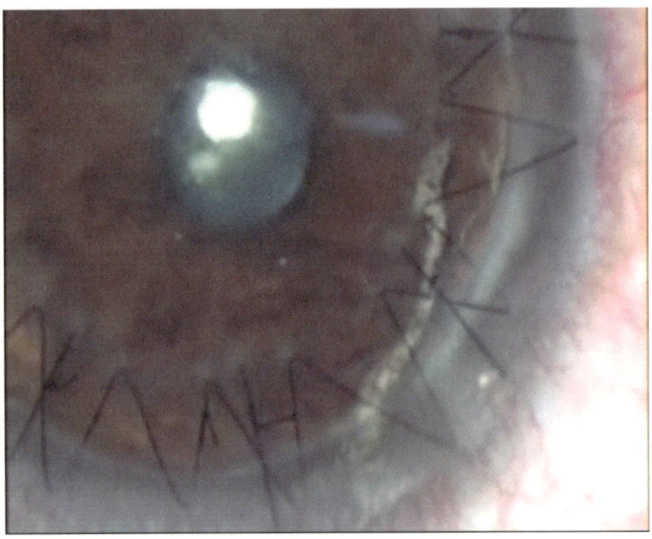

Fig. 21. One piece of sponge entraped in the donor_ host interface.

Small filaments in the interface do not affect the visual acuity even if they are located within the optical zone.

6.4 Hemorrhage in the interface

A noticeable amount of bleeding in the interface due to preexisting corneal vascularization should be managed by washing and cleaning the interface because residual blood in the interface may result in interface opacity.

6.5 Hyphema

Because the paracentesis is made in a semivertical direction to not violate the DM, introducing an instrument into the anterior chamber can cause injury to the iris tissue and hyphema (Figure 22).

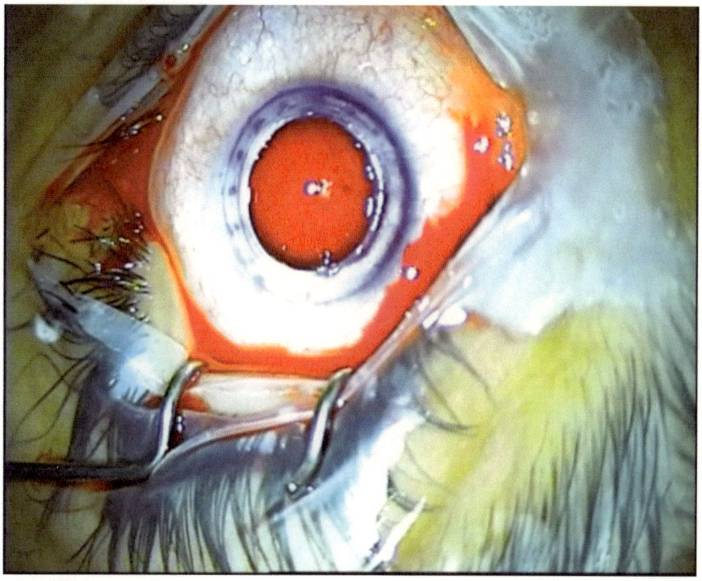

Fig. 22. Introducing surgical devices into the anterior chamber may be accompanied with hyphema.

Management includes gentle washing of the anterior chamber for flouting red blood cells after cardinal sutures are placed using a blunt-tipped cannula and irrigating the BSS through the paracentesis wound and depressing the posterior lip of the wound to drain the blood. Introducing any instrument into the anterior chamber may violate the peripheral DM and turn the condition into a major complication.

6.6 Corneal intrastromal cyst

This rare condition results from proliferation of the epithelial cells in the interface. Management includes removing donor tissue, scrapping and irrigating the recipient's bed, and performing a new graft.

6.7 Infectious keratitis

Peripheral wound infection is accompanied by edema, infiltration, loosening of sutures, and occasionally melting of the cornea. The loose sutures must be removed and placed in culture media along with suitable specimens for recognition of the etiologic organism. The treatment is similar to that for an infectious corneal ulcer. Fungal elements may cause deep ulcers without surface involvement. However, involvement of the donor—recipient interface with an infectious process requires donor tissue removal, vigorous treatment of the recipient's bed, and a new graft (Thomas & Purnell, 1965).

6.8 Allograft stromal and epithelial rejection

Stromal allograft rejection may occur after successful DALK surgeries and can be accompanied by segmental corneal edema and thickening and corneal stromal vascularization (Figure 23).

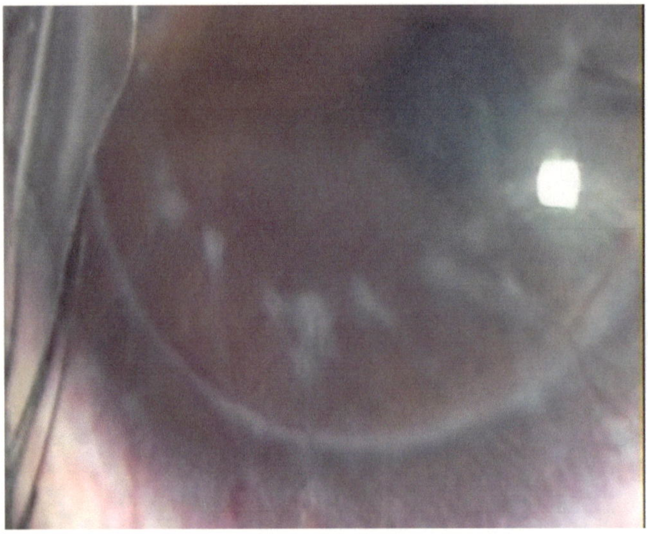

Fig. 23. Allograft corneal stromal rejection associated with vascularization and segmental corneal edema.

Epithelial allograft rejection is clinically less problematic than other types of allograft rejections. However, management includes aggressive steroid therapy to control and reverse the process. Segmental thickening of the cornea may take a long time to resolve after quiescence of the rejection process. Rarely, graft failure that requires regrafting occurs.

6.9 Persistent epithelial defect

Great attention should be focused on the tear condition, ocular surface, and lids before a patient is scheduled for corneal transplantation. Optimization of the ocular surface by lid care, lid surgery, and fornix reconstruction before attempting a corneal graft prevents delayed epithelial healing in special cases. However, management of persistent epithelial defects includes frequent nonpreserved lubricants, reduction or cessation of application of any preserved eye drop, and bandage soft contact lens. Care must be taken to recognize herpetic corneal ulceration and to treat it appropriately. In special resistant cases tarsorraphy and punctal occlusion of inferior or both puncta works well. Application of the autologous serum augments the epithelialization of the cornea. Rare unresponsive cases may lead to stromal opacification or vascularization and require regrafting.

7. Conclusion

DALK has several advantages over penetrating keratoplasty for patients with functional endothelium and a normal DM. However, many challenges tend to deter corneal surgeons from performing the procedure routinely as indicated. The advent of surgical techniques introduced by experts in corneal surgery in recent years have led to increases in DALK surgery in corneal surgical centers throughout the world. These techniques have reduced complications and the time and complexity of the procedures and increased their safety, repeatability, and efficiency. Reviewing the surgical techniques will increase our expertise in corneal surgery if we take every specific surgical "pearl" from the techniques described by experts. The expanding-bubble modification of the big-bubble technique is the one I consider most useful for routinely performing DALK surgery. I hope it will assist corneal surgeons in providing better visual results for their patients.

8. Acknowledgment

I appreciate and thank Arash Daneshgar for his technical support.

9. References

Anwar, M., & Teichmann, K.D. (2002). Deep lamellar keratoplasty. Surgical techniques for anterior lamellar keratoplasty with and without barring of Descemets membrane. *Cornea,* 21, 374-380.

Anwar, M., & Teichmann, K.D. (2002). Big-bubble technique to bare Descemet's membrane in anterior lamellar keratoplasty. *J Cataract Refract Surg,* 28, 398-403.

Arenas, A.E. (1984/1985). Deep lamellar keratoplasty dissection of host tissue with intrastromal air injection. *Cornea,* 3, 21-28.

Balestrazzi, E., Balestrazzi, A.N., Mosca, L., & Balestrazzi, A. (2002). Deep lamellar keratoplasty with trypan blue intrastromal staining. *J Cataract Refractive Surg,* 28, 929-931.

Behrooz, M.J., & Daneshgar, F. (2010) "Large-bubble" modification of the "big-bubble" technique for performing maximum depth anterior lamellar keratoplasty. *Cornea,* 29, 820–824.

Castroviejo, R. (1932). Keratoplasty. A historical and an experimental study, including a new method. Part 1. *Am J Ophthalmol,* 15, 825-838.

Daneshgar, F., & Fallahtafti, M.R. (2011). Expanding-bubble modification of the big- bubble technique for performing maximum depth anterior lamellar keratoplasty. *Eye,* 25(6), 803-8.

Hallermann, W. (1963). On the technic of lamellar keratoplasty. *Klin Monatsbl Augenheikd,* 142, 243-250.

John, T. (2004). Use of indocyanine green (ICG) and forced hydrodissection in total anterior lamellar keratoplasty (TALK). Presented at the 22nd Congress of the ESCRS, Paris, France, September 18-22, 2004.

John, T. (2006). Indocyanine green and forced hydrodissection in total anterior lamellar keratoplasty, In: *Surgical Techniques in Anterior and Posterior Lamellar Corneal Surgery,* John T., (pp. 150-164), Jaypee Brothers Medical Publishers, 81-8061-605-3, New Dehli.

Malbran, E. (1966). Lamellar keratoplasty in keratoconus. *Int Ophthalmol Clin,* 6, 99-109.

Manche, E.E., Holland, G.N., & Maloney, R.K. (1999). Deep lamellar keratoplasty using viscoelastic dissection. *Arch Ophthalmol,* 117, 1561-1565.

Melles, G.R., Lander, F., Rietveld, F.J., Remeijer, L., Beekhuis, W.H., & Binder, P.S. (1999). A new surgical technique for deep stromal, anterior lamellar keratoplasty. *Br J Ophthalmol,* 83, 327-333.

Melles, G.R.J., Remeijer, L., Geerards, A.J.M., & Beekhuis, W.H. (2000). A quick surgical technique for deep, anterior lamellar keratoplasty using visco-dissection. *Cornea,* 19, 427-432.

Morrison, J.C., & Swan, K.C. (1982). Full-thickness lamellar keratoplasty. A histopathologic study in human eyes. *Ophthalmology*, 89, 715-719.

Muhlbauer, F.X. (1842). Transplantation der cornea (Gekronte preisschrift, jas. Lindauer, Munich 1840). In: Schmidt CC, ed. Jahrbucher der in- und auslandischen gesammten medicin. Leipzig: Otto Weigand, 1842.

Reisinger, F. (1824). Die Keratoplastik Ein Versuch Zur Eiweiterung der Angenheilkunst. *Bayerische Annalen*, 1, 207-215.

Sugita, J., & Kondo, J. (1997). Deep lamellar keratoplasty with complete removal of pathological stroma for vision improvement. *Br J Ophthalmol* , 81, 184-188.

Thomas, C.L., & Purnell, E.W. (1965). Prevention and management of early and late complications of keratoplasty (penetrating and lamellar) an analysis of 120 consecutive cases. *Am J Ophthalmol*, 60, 385-405.

Von Hipple, A. (1888), *Albrecht V Graefes Arch Ophthalmol* 34, 108.

Zirm, E. (1906). Eine erfolgreiche totale keratoplastic. *Albrecht V. Graefes Arch Ophthalmol*, 64, 580.

5

Femtosecond Laser Assisted Lamellar Keratoplasties

Luigi Mosca, Laura Guccione, Luca Mosca,
Romina Fasciani and Emilio Balestrazzi
Catholic University of "Sacro Cuore" – "A. Gemelli" Polyclinic, Rome, Italy

1. Introduction

The concept of lamellar keratoplasty (LK) is that of targeted lamellar replacement of corneal tissue while retaining normal cornea. It involves replacing anterior stroma at different deepness with an anterior lamellar keratoplasty (ALK). Despite the significant advantages of LK surgery, penetrating keratoplasty (PK) remains the most common procedure, largely because lamellar surgery is more technically demanding and time consuming [1]. Moreover, interface irregularity arising from manual lamellar dissection often results in suboptimal visual outcomes [2]. Long-term graft survival rates and endothelial cell counts after PK continue to drop for many years after surgery, clearly showing the disadvantage of unnecessary replacement of a healthy endothelium in anterior-stromal disorders [3]. For these reasons, PK is now being replaced by various types of lamellar techniques that aim to replace damaged tissue only, while maintaining healthy tissue intact.
Recent improvements of surgical techniques and advances in instrumentation, such as microkeratome-assisted LK (ALTK) [4], and excimer laser assisted LK (ELLK), [5,6] have contributed to improve visual quality in corneal lamellar surgery, promoting a paradigm shift in the surgical treatment of anterior corneal disease.
The new femtosecond laser technology has been introduced for ophthalmic surgery in the last years with the aim to resolve the microkeratomes related problems in LASIK surgery [7]. This new technology has been shown to be the "top" to perform LASIK flaps, creating flaps of precise and homogeneous thickness, reducing the flap related problems (free cap, button hole, flap irregularity) and leaving more stroma for the excimer ablation allowing to correct higher refractive defects (especially with the ultrathin flaps of 90 microns).
Moreover, the femtolaser technology, allowing to perform precise corneal cuts with a planned and customized shape, offers clear advantages also applied in anterior lamellar keratoplasty (ALK) surgery[8-10].
Penetrating Keratoplasty (PK) is still the most common and effective technique for corneal transplantation, but is an "open sky" surgical technique and could be complicated by choroidal effusion or haemorrage, spontaneous lens expression and vitreous loss [1]. Moreover, this technique is characterized by an everlasting endothelial cell loss, leading to corneal decompensation necessitating a re-PK to restore a clear graft. To avoid these risks, more conservative surgical techniques have been proposed for the treatment of anterior corneal pathologies with healthy endothelium, enclosed in the great chapter of the lamellar keratoplasty (LK) [2, 3]. So that, during the last 10 years, to increase the results of traditional

manual ALK, the use of high technologic tools such as microkeratomes or excimer lasers with customized ablation patterns has been proposed, with uncertain outcomes [4-6].
With the aim to realize a more safe, repeatable and effective LK technique, suitable to every surgical skills, in 2005 we started to use the femtosecond laser technology (IntraLase, AMO, USA) (Figure 1,2) in several cases of anterior corneal pathologies (Femtolaser-assisted Anterior Lamellar Keratoplasty - Femto-ALK -. Early data published on Cornea in 2008) [9].
With the diffusion of the new manual techniques of DALK, especially the "Big Bubble" one[11-15], allowing the better visual results ever reached by a ALK, the Femto-ALK technique resulted quite inadequate. For these reasons, we developed a more effective femtolaser assisted lamellar technique: the Femtolaser-assisted Deep Anterior Lamellar Keratoplasty (Femto-DALK). Below the description of our Femtolaser-assisted LK techniques and the results reached after more than two years of follow-up with these two techniques.

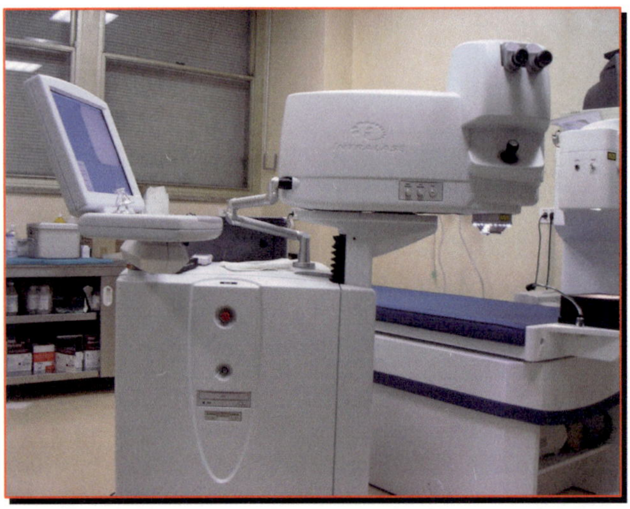

Fig. 1. The femtosecond laser (IntraLase, AMO, USA) settled near the excimer laser (Technolas 217C, Bausch & Lomb, USA) in the Laser Room of the Ophthalmic Department of Catholic University of " Sacro Cuore" of Rome, Italy.

2. Anterior Lamellar Keratoplasty (ALK)

In 2008 we published our first data on femtolaser-assisted ALK after one year of follow-up [9].
The technique of femtolaser-assisted ALK reaches modest results, with slight patient's dissatisfaction in the first months after surgery, even if after complete suture removal the visual acuity resulted drastically growing up (Figure 3). Nevertheless, these initial results were not validated by a longer follow-up. Below, we present the clinical results more than three years postoperatively.

2.1 Clinical experience with Femto-ALK

The experience performing Anterior Lamellar Keratoplasty (ALK) for different corneal pathologies starts in May 2005, first with a 15 kHz (10 cases) and then with a 60kHz (11 cases) femtosecond laser (IntraLase, AMO, USA). From July 2005 to December 2007 has been performed 21 consecutive femtolaser-assisted ALK (Femto-ALK) procedures for different corneal pathologies (5 post-traumatic corneal scar, 3 post-keratitis corneal leucoma, and 13 moderate keratoconus).

2.2 Femtosecond laser features

The femtosecond laser of the Ophthalmic Department of Catholic University of "Sacro Cuore" (Figure 1) features are as follows: spot size of < 3μm, repetition rate of 60 kHz (for the first 10 patients the repetition rate was 15kHz); laser pulse duration of 600-800 fs (±50); maximum laser pulse peak power of 12 MW (±2); central laser wavelength of 1053nm; maximum pulse energy of 7.3 mJ (±0.7); maximum laser beam output of 110mW (±11). The laser acts with four different ablation patterns (Raster, double raster, spiral and pocket) that can be mixed by the surgeon for the surgical target. The femtosecond laser pulses result in multiple corneal intrastromal gas bubbles (micro-cavitations), requiring only a manual light lamellar dissection using a blunted spatula, to create the intrastromal cut with a smooth surface.

2.3 Surgical procedure

The Femto-ALK surgical technique has been realized in two surgical steps:
The first step was performed in the laser room where a femtosecond laser cut was created on both donor and receiving cornea(Figure 2). In the second step, performed in the surgery room, the donor lamella was sutured into the receiving stromal bed with 16 radial 10/0 nylon stitches.
To realize the donor lamella, the cut was performed on an entire donor cornea, analyzed and delivered by an ocular tissue bank, positioned on an artificial anterior chamber (Moria, France). Mean lamellar diameter was 8.34mm ± 0.28 SD (range: 8.2 - 8.7mm), and mean lamellar thickness was 353.91μm ± 38.82SD (range: 220 - 400μm). The donor button has been planned thicker than the amount of receiving cornea removed, in way to restore a normal corneal thickness (at least 550 micron), and 0.2 mm larger, in way to avoid too much corneal compression with the sutures and to evade the risk of anterior chamber (AC) reduction after surgery.

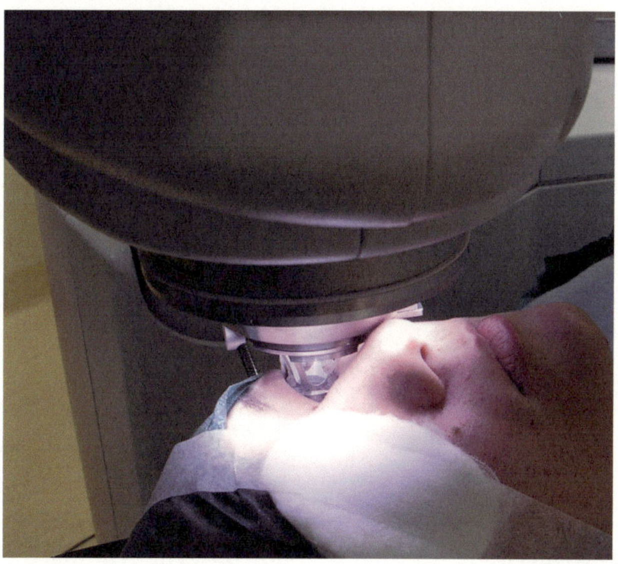

Fig. 2. Femtosecond laser cut on recipient bed after docking on the cornea of the patient.

Under topical anaesthesia (Ossibuprocaine 4% drops for 4 times), a disposable suction ring was positioned at the sclero-limbal margin to stabilize the eye. After the docking, the femtosecond laser cut (Figure 2) on receiving corneal stroma was performed to leave at least 200μm residual stromal bed (mean stromal cut deepness of 243.91μm ±51.59SD, with a mean diameter of 8.13mm ±0.37 SD, and mean residual stromal bed of 181.61μm ± 57.78SD).
After stromal laser cut execution, the patient was carried in the surgery room where the corneal button was removed with a blunt spatula leaving the clear stromal residual bed. Then, the donor lamella was first secured in the recipient bed with four 10/0 nylon cardinal sutures at the 6, 12, 9 and 3 o'clock positions, and subsequently it was sutured with twelve more 10/0 nylon radial stitches. Intraoperatively, corneal astigmatism was evaluated with a corneal disposable keratometer, (Janach, Como, Italy) and suture adjustment, if required, was performed. At the end of surgery, a soft contact lens was placed on the eye surface to help restoring of corneal epithelium. Topical antibiotics (Nethylmicine), steroids (Desamethasone 0.18%) and artificial tear drops (Hyaluronate sodium 0.2%) were applied several times a day, and then tapered and titrated, basing on the corneal transparency and scarring of the surgical wound.
The surgical plannings have been realized in all cases basing on the accurate preoperative pachymetric values found with optical pachymetry (Confoscan 4, Nidek technologies, Tokyo, Japan; and Orbscan II, Bausch & Lomb, CA, USA).
In all the cases performed, the surgery restored a clear cornea from the first week after surgery with an interface hard to detect at the slit lamp examination.
The postoperative corneal thickness (mean corneal pachymetry: 542.48μm ± 33.20SD), curvature (mean K reading: 44.32D ± 13.50SD) and shape resulted nearer to physiologic values. Nevertheless, the results in visual acuity obtained with the Femto-ALK were not so brilliant as planned, especially in the keratoconic eyes, with a very slow recovery time. Three months after surgery, mean BSCVA was 0.30, increasing to 0.40 after complete suture removal six months later, and stabilizing 12 months postoperatively to 0.64 (the Figure 3 showed the BSCVA during follow-up).

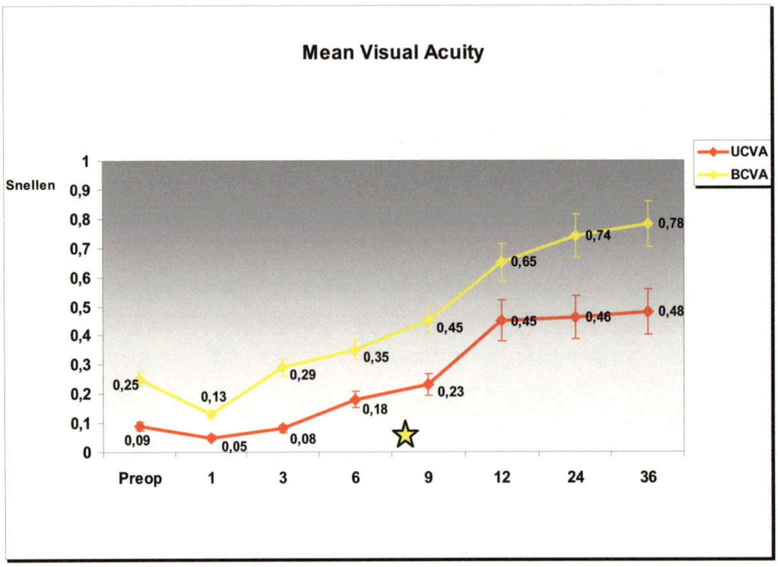

Fig. 3. Visual acuity results three years after Femto-ALK. The yellow star marks the mean removal suture period.

Analyzing all our cases with the confocal microscopy analysis (Confoscan4), we found that this unsatisfactory visual results were mostly related to the excessive thickness of residual stromal bed (150 microns or more), resulting in a irregular stromal interface (Fig. 4) with dark folds before suture removal (published on "Cornea 2008 Jul; 27(6): 668-72"); few months after suture removal, these findings disappeared gradually with a parallel increase of the BSCVA, setting to 0.64 Snellen at 12 months of follow-up. At two years of follow up the mean BSCVA resulted increased to 0.74 ± 0.18SD. After a three years of follow-up, these visual results resulted quite similar (mean UCVA of 0.48 ± 0.13SD and mean BSCVA of 0.78 ± 0.13SD), confirming the stability of the outcomes during time and the validity of the Femto-ALK technique (Figure 3) and confirming that, comparing to penetrating keratoplasty (PK), lamellar keratoplasty need more time to stabilize the results.

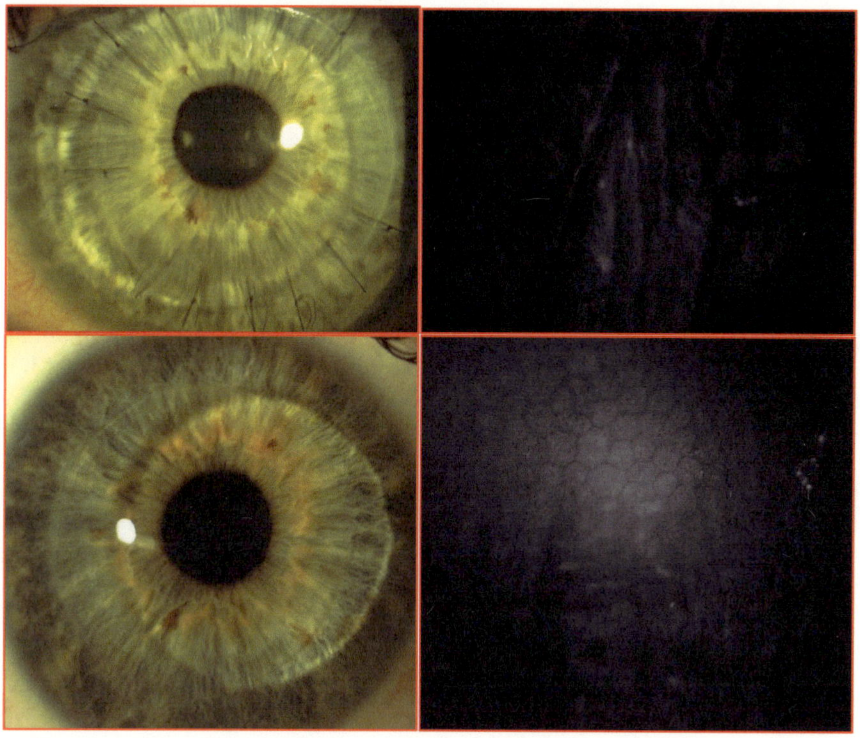

Fig. 4. Femto-ALK results: a. slit lamp examination 3 months after surgery shows a clear graft with sutures still on; b. Confoscan 4 confocal microscopy analysis at three months shows dark folds of the residual bed stroma related to the slow visual recovery; c. Six months postoperatively slit lamp shows a clear graft and confocal analysis (d) shows disappearance of the stromal folds and a healthy endothelium.

3. Deep Anterior Lamellar Keratoplasty (DALK)

After the quite unsatisfactory results obtained with the Femto-ALK technique, in keratoconic cases, We designed a new surgical technique trying to duplicate the superior results obtained with the descemetic and pre-descemetic DALK techniques: the femtolaser-assisted DALK.

Deep Anterior Lamellar Keratoplasty (DALK) has the target of removing all the pathological stromal tissue, maintaining only the Descemet/endothelium layers in the recipient bed,

replacing it with a healthy stromal tissue, and restoring in that way a normal corneal thickness and shape [11-13]. However, there are some drawbacks to DALK, including the great difficulty of the manual intrastromal dissection and the fact that the procedure rarely achieves precision, resulting in low visual acuity and poor optical quality, especially if Descemet's membrane is not reached with the Big Bubble technique. There is also a high risk of micro- or macro-perforation [13-15], often requiring a conversion to Penetrating Keratoplasty. Many of these problems could be focused by the femtosecond laser assisted deep anterior lamellar keratoplasty (femto-DALK) procedure created to open this difficult surgery to every surgical skills.
In keratoconus patients, the goal is to utilise a surgical option that could be compared in results to manual descemetic DALK, preserving the health and integrity of the corneal endothelium layer.

3.1 Clinical experience with Femto-DALK

This technique was performed on 21 eyes of 21 patients, with advanced keratoconus with a mean corneal power of 53.2D ± 6.08SD and a mean corneal topographic astigmatism of 4.3D ± 2.82SD. Mean UCVA was 0.1 ± 0.05SD, and mean BSCVA was 0.33 ± 0.15SD; mean SE was -3.73 ± 2.65SD, and mean preoperative pachymetry was 361.19µm ±46.85SD.

3.2 Surgical procedure

The new technique of DALK assisted by a femtosecond laser has been planned in two surgical phases.
During the first phase, performed in the laser room, a deep 8.2mm wide stromal cut on receiving bed is performed with a 60 kHz femtosecond laser (IntraLase, AMO, USA), leaving at least 100µm of residual stromal bed, on the base of the pachymetric parameters of the patient (optical pachymetry evaluated by Orbscan II). Then, a +4 D spherical hyperopic PRK ablation with an optical zone of 6.5 mm (8.5 mm of maximum ablation diameter), to reduce the peripheral bed thickness in the way to reach a more uniform stromal bed thickness, followed by a 40-60 µm, 7.0mm wide, PTK ablation with fluid mask to reach as much as possible the Descemet's layer, is carried out with an excimer laser (Technolas 217C, B&L, USA) on the residual stromal bed (Fig. 5).

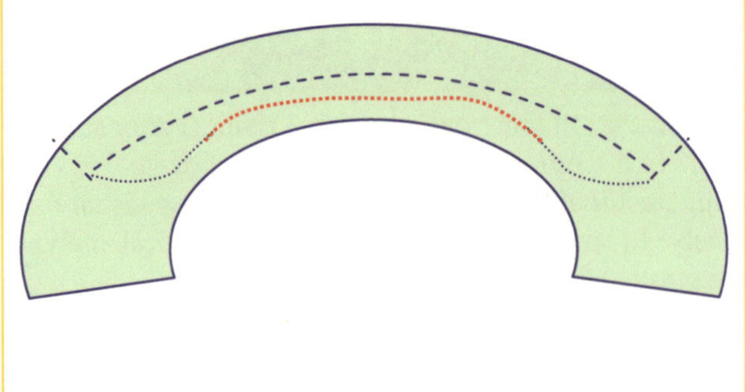

Fig. 5. First step of Femto-DALK technique: preparation of recipient bed in the laser room: ("----") Femtosecond laser cut as deep as possible, leaving at least 100microns of stromal residual bed; ("….") Excimer laser ablation +3/4 sph PRK to reduce peripheral bed thickness; ("….") Excimer laser 40-60 microns PTK to reach Descemet/epithelium layer as near as possible.

In the second surgical phase, performed in the operatory room, the donor button is cut from an entire cornea delivered by an Italian Corneal Bank with a corneal trephine (Hanna suction system, Moria, France) 0.25mm wider than the receiving bed (Fig. 6); then, after Descemet/endothelium layers manual stripping, the donor button is sutured on receiving stromal bed using 16 radial 10/0 nylon stitches.

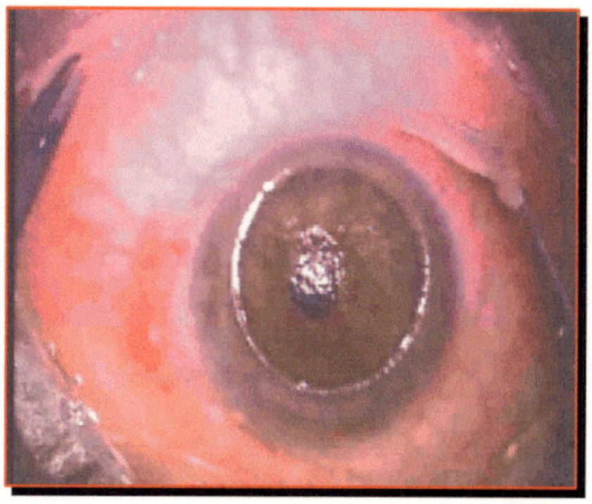

Fig. 6. Second step of Femto-DALK technique in operatory room: Suturing of the donor lamella after Descemet/endothelium layer manual stripping on recipient bed with 16 radial nylon stitches.

During the surgical procedure, two patients experienced a perforation performing the receiving bed cut with the femtolaser, that required a conversion to PK.
In another case, a microperforation occurred during the PTK ablation, that was managed with air injection in AC, and then the procedure was carried out without any further complication in operatory room.
One week after surgery a clear graft is shown in all cases, with an interface very hard to detect at slit lamp examination (Fig. 7). In all patients, one month after surgery the mean BSCVA was 0.40, three months later was 0.60, and at the one-year follow-up mark a clear graft and a regular astigmatism was reached (Figure 8), and BSCVA resulted 0.74. Two years after surgery, all patients experience stable results in both UCVA (0.43 ± 0.25SD) and BSCVA (0.84 ± 0.13SD), showing the validity of this femtolaser assisted DALK technique (Figure 9).

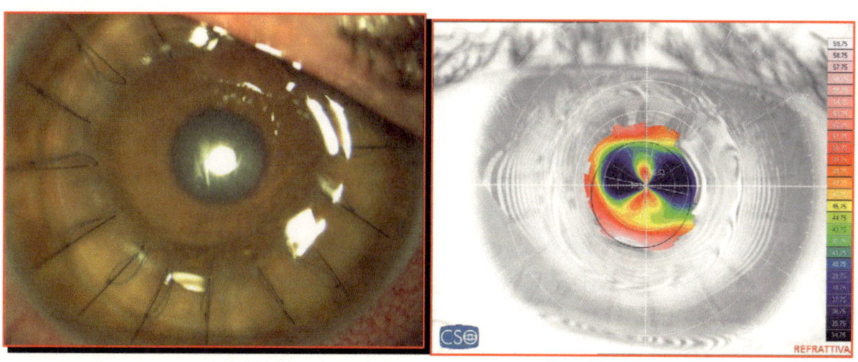

Fig. 7. Slit lamp examination (on left) at first week shows a clear graft with 16 radial nylon stitches; the topography analysis shows a regular "with the rule" astigmatism.

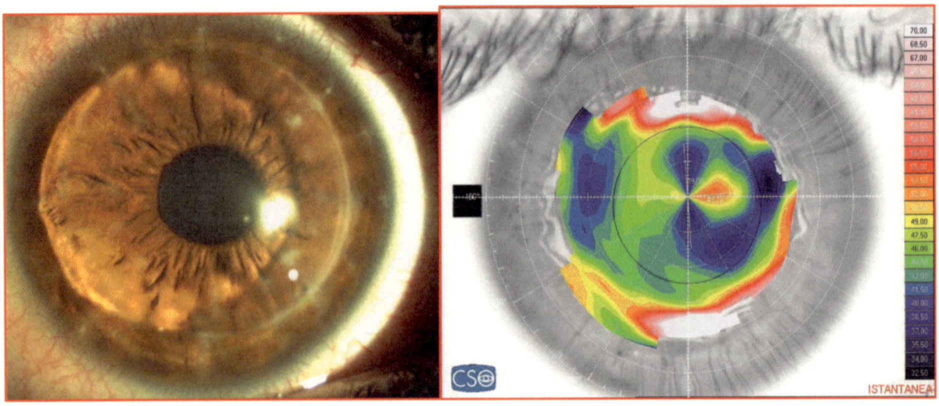

Fig. 8. Slit lamp examination (on the left) at 12 months shows a clear graft after all sutures removal. The topography analysis (on the right) shows a regular bow-tie "against the rule" astigmatism.

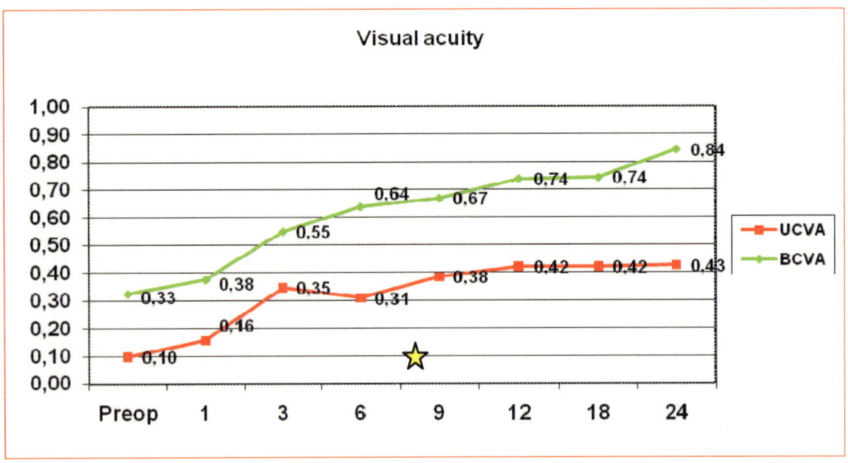

(the yellow star marks the mean suture removal period)

Fig. 9. Visual acuity results of Femto-DALK after 2 years (Mean follow-up : 32.94 months ±11,50SD)

Postoperative optical pachymetry evaluation with Optical Coherence Tomography (Visante, Carl Zeiss, Jena, Germany) and Confoscan4 showed a mean residual stromal bed thickness of 67.19µm ± 13.19 SD (range: 50 to 85 micron), three months after surgery (Fig.10).

In three cases of our case series, a stromal rejection of the donor lamella occurred at 5, 16 and 18 months after surgery. The stromal reject was resolved in all cases only with topical steroid therapy (Fig. 11). Confocal microscopy analysis with Confoscan4 showed no recipient endothelium involvement, oedema of deep donor lamellar stroma, immunological infiltrates of the anterior stroma of donor lamella, and inflammatory infiltrates and oedema of epithelium of the graft (Fig. 12).

The case observed 5 months after surgery developed four months later an herpetic keratitis of the donor lamella and was removed from the study after nine months of follow-up.

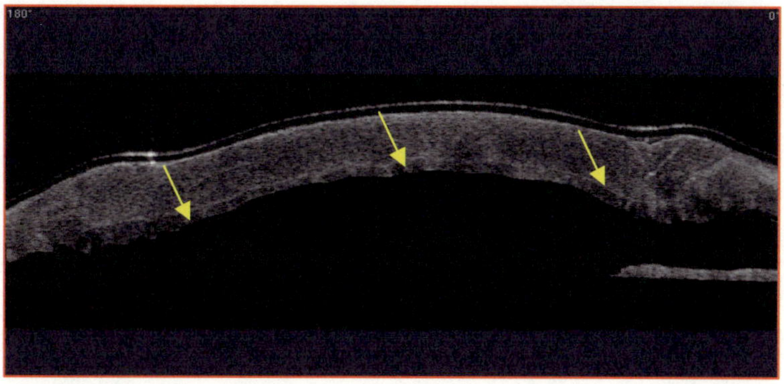

Fig. 10. Optical Coherence Tomography of a Femto-DALK shows a regular residual bed thickness 1 month after surgery (the yellow arrows mark the residual stromal bed).

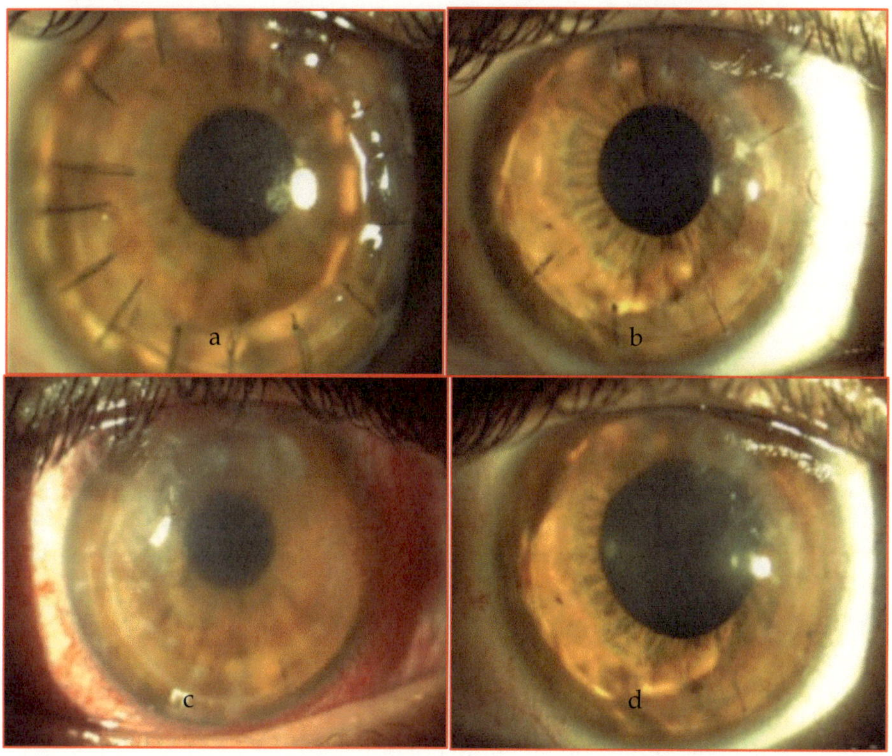

Fig. 11. Case of stromal reject 15 months after surgery: a. Clear graft two weeks after surgery; b. Clear graft before all suture removal nine months after surgery; c. Stromal rejection 15 months postoperatively with neovessels and massive stromal oedema; d. Complete resolution of the stromal rejection after two weeks of massive topical steroid therapy.

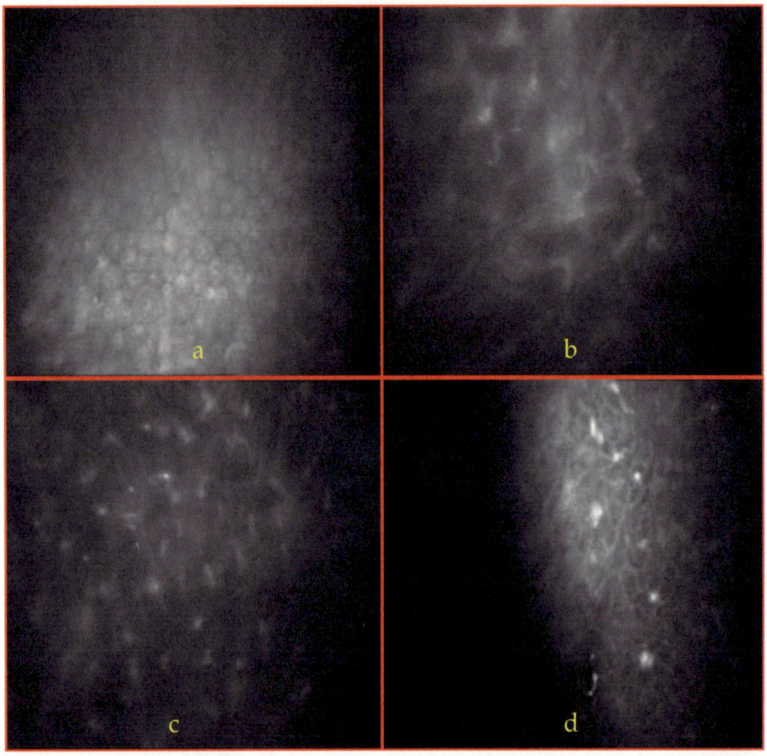

Fig. 12. Confoscan 4 confocal microscopy analysis of graft rejection of Femto-DALK: a. no recipient endothelium involvement, b. oedema of deep donor lamellar stroma; c. immunological infiltrates of the anterior stroma of donor lamella; d. inflammatory infiltrates and oedema of epithelium of the graft

4. Posterior Lamellar Keratoplasty Techniques (DSEK/DLEK)

4.1 Clinical experience with Femto-DSEK/DLEK

Another application of the femtosecond laser technology is the new frontier of lamellar surgery: the posterior lamellar keratoplasty (PLK).

The new technique of Descemet Stripping Endothelial Keratoplasty (DSEK)[16, 17] assisted by a femtosecond laser has been planned to perform more regular and precise endothelial donor buttons.

We performed this femtosecond-assisted DSEK technique on 12 eyes of 12 patients using the original "taco" technique for endothelial lamella insertion.

4.2 Surgical procedure

The donor lamella is performed on an entire donor cornea delivered by an Italian Corneal Bank using an artificial anterior chamber (Moria, France) and the 60kHz femtosecond laser with a double raster pattern of 9mm diameter at 400 microns of depth. Then, the button is punched with a 8.50mm diameter corneal trephine and the two resulting lamellae are divided with forceps (Figure 13). The receiving bed is prepared in the usual way with endothelium/Descemet layer manual stripping. Then, the donor button is inserted in AC with the "taco" technique and settled in place with air injection.

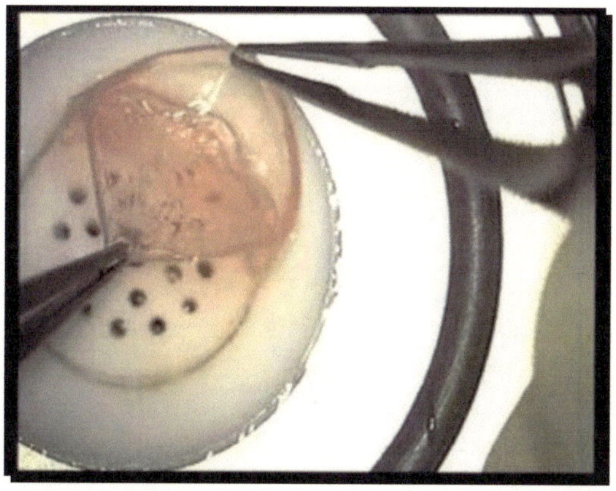

Fig. 13. Preparing the donor lamella: division the two lamellae with forceps after donor corneal punch.

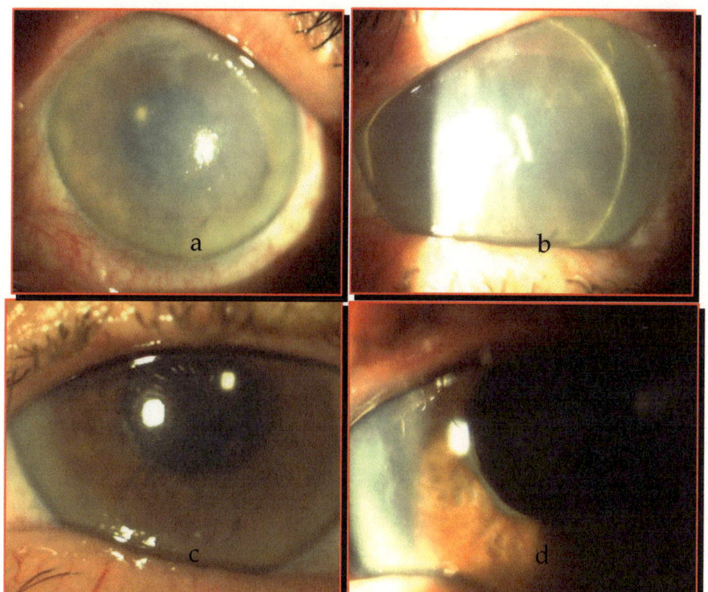

Fig. 14. Clinical case of Femto-DSEK (with "taco" technique): Preoperative slit lamp examination shows massive corneal oedema (a); One week postoperative shows corneal oedema, endothelial lamella centred with air in AC (b); one month postoperatively the corneal oedema is reduced (c) and three months postoperatively a clear graft is shown (d)

One day postoperatively, the donor lamella resulted in place in 9 cases (Figure 14). In three cases, the donor lamella resulted dislocated (Fig. 15), requiring a second air injection in AC to reposition it back.

One month after surgery the BSCVA resulted not so good (mean BSCVA 0.5 ± 0.15 SD) and increased slowly during the follow-up, resulting a little bit higher six months after surgery (0.58 ± 0.23SD).

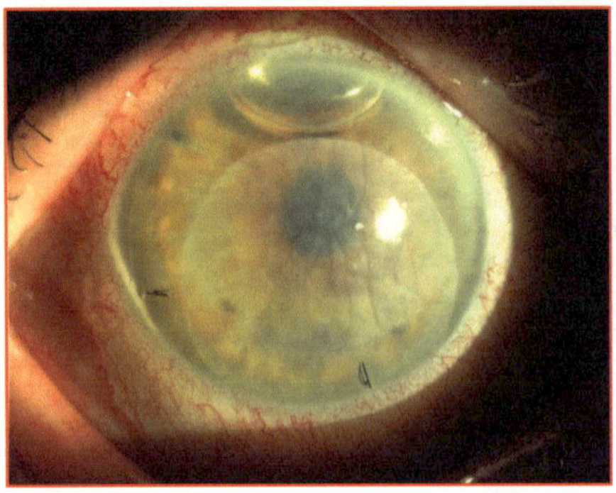

Fig. 15. Donor lamella dislocated downward three days after surgery.

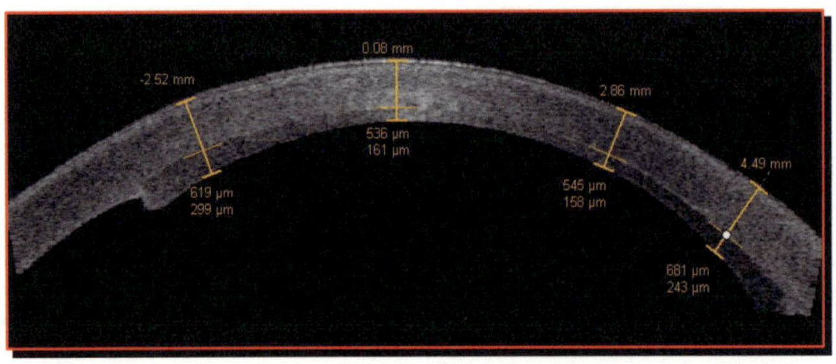

Fig. 16. Optical Coherence Tomography with Visante shows the endothelial lamellar thickness.

To assess the precision, safety and reproducibility of femtosecond laser cut we studied the donor lamellae with a Spectral Domain Optical Coherent Tomography analysis (Visante, Carl Zeiss Meditec, Jena, Germany). The planned donor lamellar thickness of 198µm ± 25.45SD (range 190-210), resulted 177µm ± 34.50SD (range 150-200) three months after surgery (Fig. 16). These results probably were related to the deswelling of the donor lamella during the follow-up.

Nevertheless, the greatest problem using the "taco" technique was the high surgical endothelial cell loss. In fact, with Confoscan 4 confocal microscopy analysis we found that endothelial cell loss was around 49% three months after surgery (preoperative mean ECD: 2389 ± 368 cell/mm2 (range: 2150-2580; postoperative mean ECD: 1028 ± 582 cell/mm2 (range 787-1550), with respect to the 22% of PK procedures. These higher rate resulted in a high graft failure percentage (around 55%).

For this reason, we began to utilize the "pull in technique" with the Busin folder. Utilizing this new device to insert the donor lamella, we performed the Femto-DSEK in 12 eyes of 10 patients with endothelial pathologies. With this technique, intraoperative endothelial cell loss resulted around 30%, with better postoperative results (Figure17). During the follow-up, two cases required endothelial lamella replacing and two cases required a penetrating keratoplasty after the DSEK failure for vision recovery.

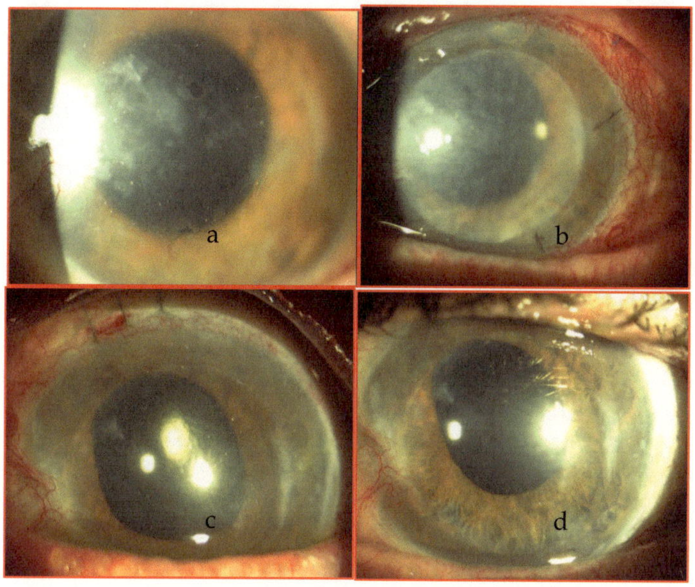

Fig. 17. Clinical case of Femto-DSEK (with Busin folder): Preoperative massive corneal oedema with bullous keratopathy (a); one week postoperatively the donor lamella is well adherent but corneal oedema is still present (b); One month postoperatively endothelial lamella is well centred and adherent with light corneal oedema (c); three months postoperatively there's a clear cornea and the BSCVA results 0.7 (d).

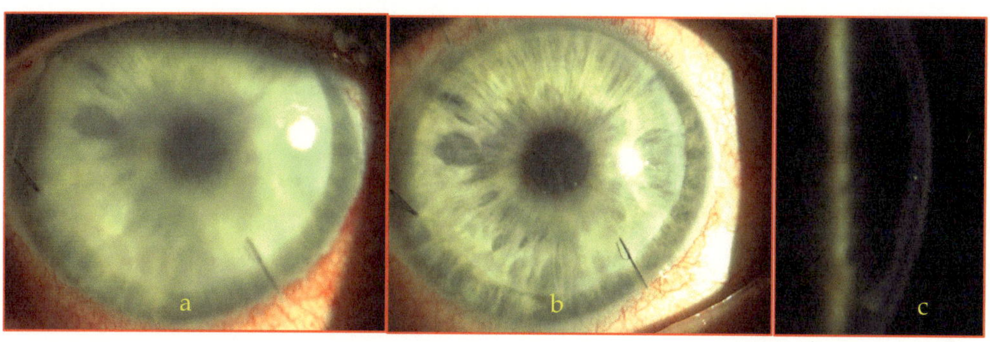

Fig. 18. Femto-DSEK: a. one week after surgery stromal oedema is still present; b. one month postoperatively a clear graft with little oedema well centred and strongly adherent to the internal surface but with the "step" between donor and recipient (c)

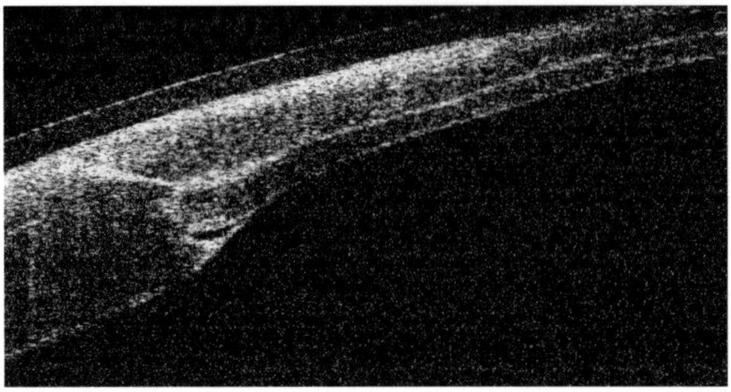

Fig. 19. Optical Coherent Tomography (on the left) of Femto-DLEK shows perfect "matching" of donor lamella like an "insert" into the recipient bed.

To avoid the problems of the endothelial lamellar dislocation (Figure 15) and the presence of the "step" between donor and recipient (Figure 18), we tried to perform a Femto-DLEK technique (basing on the Melles' manual DLEK technique) using the femtosecond laser to perform the endothelial lamellar cut both in the donor cornea and the recipient one [18]. In this way we tried to realize a perfect "match" between donor and recipient cornea with the donor lamella "inserted" in the recipient bed (Figure. 19), but the stroma-stroma interface resulted in a hard scarring showing low visual results (0.3 or little more) with patient dissatisfaction that required a PK and we abandoned this technique.

5. Conclusions

Both the femtolaser assisted ALK and DALK techniques seem to be effective in restoring a clear and normal cornea with a good recovery one year after surgery with a mean BSCVA of 0.60 and 0.80, respectively. The Femto-DALK technique resulted more rapid in recovery time and more effective with results comparable to the manual descemetic DALK technique.

With the new femtosecond lasers machines developed by different manufacturers, femtolaser-assisted Anterior Lamellar Keratoplasties will be available to more surgeons.

The development of the femtosecond laser softwares and the possible association with scanning topography systems could help in performing customized treatment to the single cornea, improving the results reached with the empirical femtolaser-assisted ALK techniques.

Moreover, femtosecond laser allows to perform precise lamellar thickness graft for posterior lamellar keratoplasty. This application of the femtosecond laser showed good results especially associated with the Busin folder "pull-in" technique.

The femtosecond laser showed to be a dynamic surgical tool, enabling surgeons to perform safe and reproducible anterior and posterior lamellar keratoplasty procedures.

Nevertheless, we must be cautious in the application of this exciting technology, remembering that it is still "a work in progress" and the preliminary results need to be evaluated by longer follow-up.

6. References

[1] Laibson P R. Current concepts and techniques in corneal transplantation. Curr Opin in Ophth 2002; 13: 220-223.

[2] Tan DT, Mehta JS. Future directions in lamellar corneal transplantation. Cornea. 2007 Oct; 26 (9 Suppl 1): S21-8.

[3] Malbran E, Malbran E J, Malvran J. Lamellar keratoplasty in keratoconus. Ophthalmology 2001; 108 (6): 1010.

[4] Busin M, Zambianchi L, Arffa RC. Microkeratome-assisted lamellar keratoplasty for the surgical treatment of keratoconus. Ophthalmology. 2005 Jun;112(6):987-97.

[5] Buratto L, Belloni S, Valeri R. Excimer laser lamellar keratoplasty of augmented thickness for keratoconus. J Refract Surg 1998 Sep-Oct; 14 (5): 517-525.

[6] Spadea L, Giammaria D, Fiasca A, Verrecchia V.Excimer laser-assisted lamellar keratoplasty for the surgical treatment of keratoconus. J Cataract Refract Surg. 2009 Jan;35(1):105-12

[7] Ratkay-Traub I, Ferincz IE, Juhasz T, Kurtz RM, Krueger RR. First clinical results with the femtosecond neodynium-glass laser in refractive surgery. J Refract Surg. 2003 Mar-Apr;19(2):94-103.

[8] Nurozler MO. Femtosecond laser holds promise for lamellar keratoplasty applications. ESCRS Eurotimes, vol 10, May 2005.

[9] Mosca L, Fasciani R, Tamburelli C, Buzzonetti L, Guccione L, Mandarà E, Balestrazzi E. Femtosecond laser-assisted lamellar keratoplasty: early results. Cornea. 2008 Jul;27(6):668-72.

[10] Ehrenhaus MP, Aliprandis E, Lazzaro DR. Sizing guidelines for performing lamellar keratoplasty with the Intralase femtosecond laser. Invest Ophthalmol Vis Sci 2006; 47: E-Abstract 3594.

[11] Fontana L, Parente G, Tassinari G. Clinical outcomes after deep anterior lamellar keratoplasty using the big-bubble technique in patients with keratoconus. Am J Ophthalmol. 2007 Jan;143(1):117-124. Epub 2006 Oct 20.

[12] Fournié P, Coullet J, Moalic S, Malecaze F, Chapotot E, Arné JL. Deep anterior lamellar keratoplasty in the surgical treatment of keratoconus. A 1-year follow-up. J Fr Ophtalmol. 2006 Jun;29(6):602-13.

[13] Noble BA, Agrawal A, Collins C, Saldana M, Brogden PR, Zuberbuhler B. Deep Anterior Lamellar Keratoplasty (DALK): visual outcome and complications for a heterogeneous group of corneal pathologies. Cornea. 2007 Jan;26(1):59-64.

[14] Shimmura S, Tsubota K.Deep anterior lamellar keratoplasty. Curr Opin Ophthalmol. 2006 Aug;17(4):349-55.

[15] Balestrazzi E, Mosca L, Balestrazzi A. "Descemet's membrane dyeing technique" in Atlas of Lamellar Keratoplasty. Fabiano Ed, 2007.

[16] Melles GRJ, LanderF, Dooren BTH. Preliminary clinical results of posterior lamellar keratoplasty through a sclerocorneal pocket incision. Ophthalmology 2000; 107: 1850-1857.

[17] Terry MA, Ousley PJ, Will B. A practical femtosecond laser procedure for DLEK endothelial transplantation: cadaver eye histology and topography. Cornea. 2005 May;24(4): 453-9.

[18] Mehta JS, Shilbayeh R, Por YM, Cajucom-Uy H, Beuerman RW, Tan DT. Femtosecond laser creation of donor ornea buttons for Descemet-stripping endothelial keratoplasty. J Cataract Refract Surg. 2008 Nov;34(11):1970-5

6

Descemet's Stripping with Automated Endothelial Keratoplasty (DSAEK) in Patients with Black Diaphragm Intraocular (BDI) Lens

Hui-Jin Chen, Yan-sheng Hao and Jing Hong
Department of Ophthalmology, Peking University Third Hospital, Beijing, China

1. Introduction

A stable anterior chamber is a crucial factor to DSAEK. In aniridic patients with BDI lens, the anterior and posterior segment has direct communication at the periphery of the BDI lens. Maintenance of the air bubble in the anterior chamber would be problematic. Pressure equilibrium must be established on both sides of the BDI lens before the air bubble is introduced into the anterior chamber.

Compared with traditional full-thickness keratoplasty, endothelial keratoplasty (EK) is a great breakthrough for the treatment of corneal endothelial disorders because this new technique maintains a more regular corneal anterior surface, preserves more corneal biomechanical tensile strength and provides more rapid visual rehabilitation. Descemet's stripping with automated endothelial keratoplasty (DSAEK) is currently most favored procedure of EK, in which the donor disc dissection was performed with an automated microkeratome that allows smoother interface and more accurate control of graft thickness.

A stable iris-lens diaphragm is essential to intraoperative donor unfolding and maintenance of air in the anterior chamber, and thus a critical factor for DSAEK. Although it was once considered as a relative contraindication, DSAEK has begun to be undertaken in patients in whom the iris-lens diaphragm was anatomically or functionally abnormal.[1,2,3]

In the past decade, patients with aniridia and aphakia/cataract were treated with black diaphragm intraocular (BDI) lens which is composed of a central optic surrounded by a black diaphragm and 2 haptics. This lens could alleviate the patients' symptom of glare and photophobia and increase vision. However, this BDI lens differs from the natural iris-lens diaphragm for more rigidity and less compliance. Besides, the chamber anterior to the BDI lens has direct communication with the vitreous cavity at the gap between the diaphragm and haptics of the lens. Difficulties may be encountered in maintaining the air bubble in the anterior chamber. Herein, we present 3 consecutive cases of bullous keratopathy with BDI lens who underwent DSAEK, the etiologies included 1 congenital aniridia and 2 traumatic iris loss.

2. Case report

2.1 Case 1

A 50-year-old man present with bullous keratopathy in his left eye. He had a history of left corneal laceration in 2000, and underwent black diaphragm intraocular (BDI) lens implantation in 2003. Ophthalmic examination revealed a linear corneal scar, the majority of iris was absent except the nasal remnants adhering to the corneal endothelium. Ultrasound biomicroscopy (UBM) showed that the BDI lens was in the right position. Preoperative best-corrected visual acuity in the left was counting fingers, and the intraocular pressure (IOP)

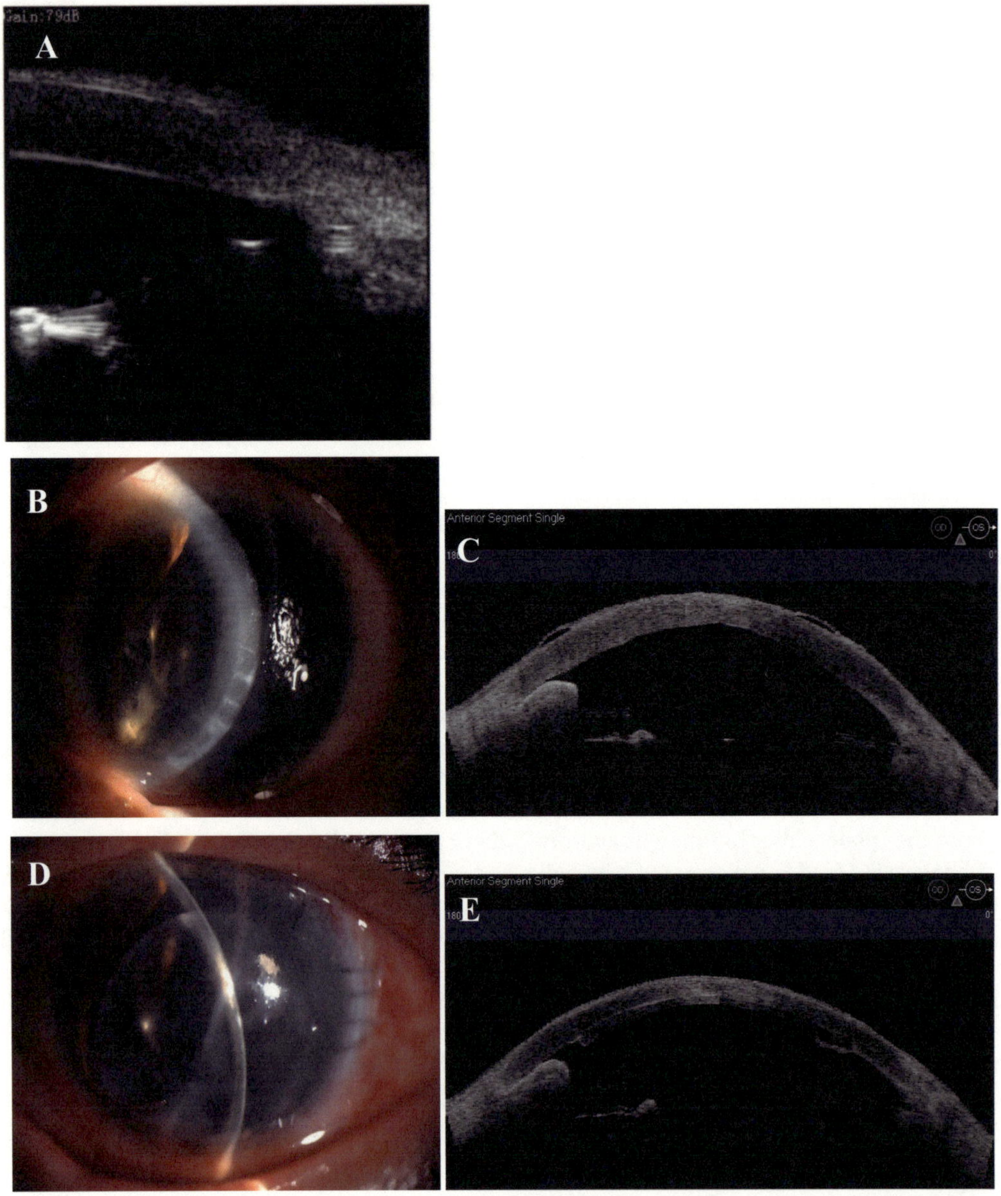

Fig. 1. (case 1) UBM shows that BDI lens is at the right position of ciliary sulcus (A). Preoperative slit lamp photograph shows edematous cornea (B). AS-OCT shows bullea of the epithelium.The nasal iris remnant is adherent to the cornea (C). Postoperative slit lamp photograph (D) and AS-OCT (E) shows a well apposed graft.

was controlled within normal limit with medication. DSAEK was uneventful. However, on the first postoperative day the upper part of the graft was observed detached and the air bubble was invisible in the anterior chamber. Graft reattachment surgery was performed. The eye was first inflated to the normal pressure with balanced salt solution (BSS) that was injected into both the vitreous cavity and the anterior chamber. After that, the anterior chamber was inserted with 0.15ml viscoelastic (Healon GV) followed by filtered air bubble. The patient was instructed to maintain a face-up position for at least 4 hours. The graft was successfully reattached after this procedure. Anterior segment optical coherence tomography (AS-OCT, Visante; Carl Zeiss Meditec, Dublin, California) showed a well apposed graft. The left eye increased to 0.3. The IOP was normal postoperatively. But it rose to 43mmHg around one month postoperatively. It was controlled to normal by medically.

2.2 Case 2

A 49-year-old woman present with DSAEK in her left eye, as history of bilateral congenital aniridia and cataract and lens implantation in 2002. On examination, pendular nystagmus. Preoperative best-corrected visual acuity was 0.12 in the right and 0.1 in the left, and the IOP was 17 mmHg in the right and 20mmHg in the left when using eye-drops. The left cornea

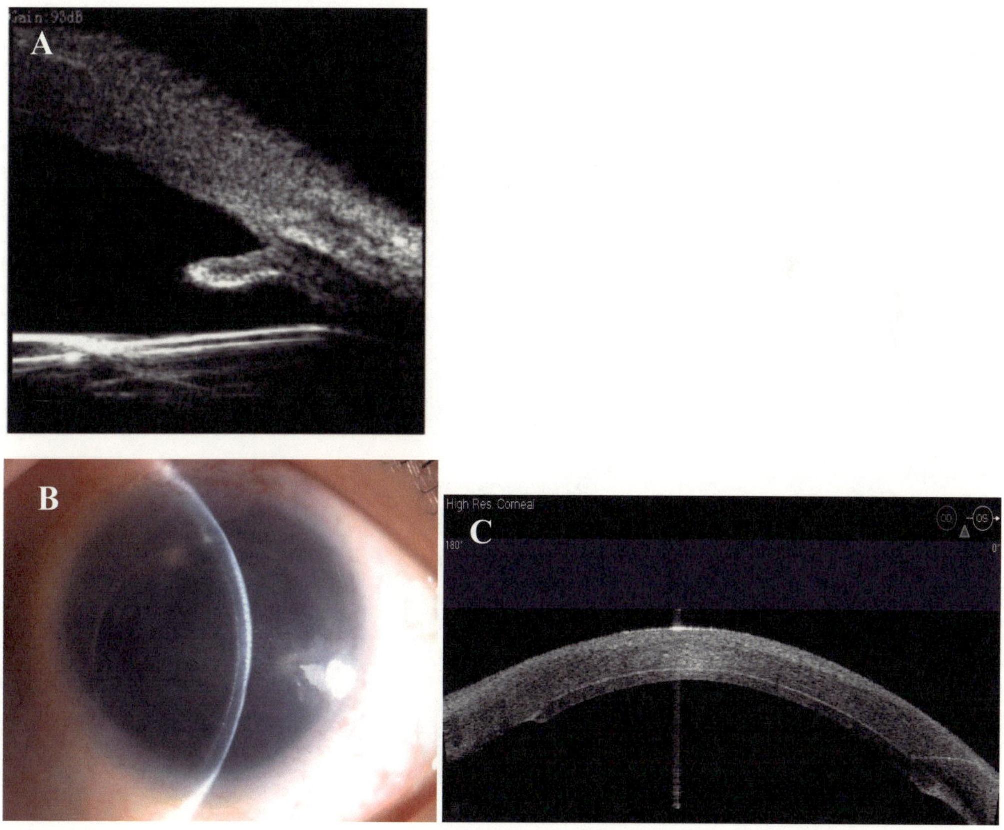

Fig. 2. (case 2) UBM shows iris remnants at periphery. The BDI lens is at the right position of ciliary sulcus (A). Postoperative slit lamp photograph (B) and AS-OCT (C) shows a well apposed graft.

had a ground glass appearance. UBM showed that the BDI lens was in the right position. The lens was sutured. DSAEK was uneventful. 1 month after DSAEK, the patient suffered an ocular hypertony that couldn't be controlled by medication. Ciliary body photocoagulation was undertaken to lower the IOP. The last follow-up visit was 2 month after DSAEK, her IOP was 12 mmHg, and visual acuity was 0.12.

2.3 Case 3

A 79-year-old man present with bullous keratopathy in his right eye. He underwent traumatic cataract extraction and BDI lens implantation in 2003. On examination, his best-corrected visual acuity was hand motion in the right, and the IOP was within the normal limits without medication. DSAEK was performed using a neonate donor. The graft markedly contracted during the first postoperative week. Two months later, the patient received a second surgery to exchange the graft. No postoperative complications occurred this time. The last follow-up visit was 3 month after the second DSAEK, the visual acuity improved to 0.1. IOP was good.

The DSAEK basic procedures were same with the reported by Terry. The implants was prepared by using a Moria (Antony, France) automated microkeratome and a Moria artificial chamber.

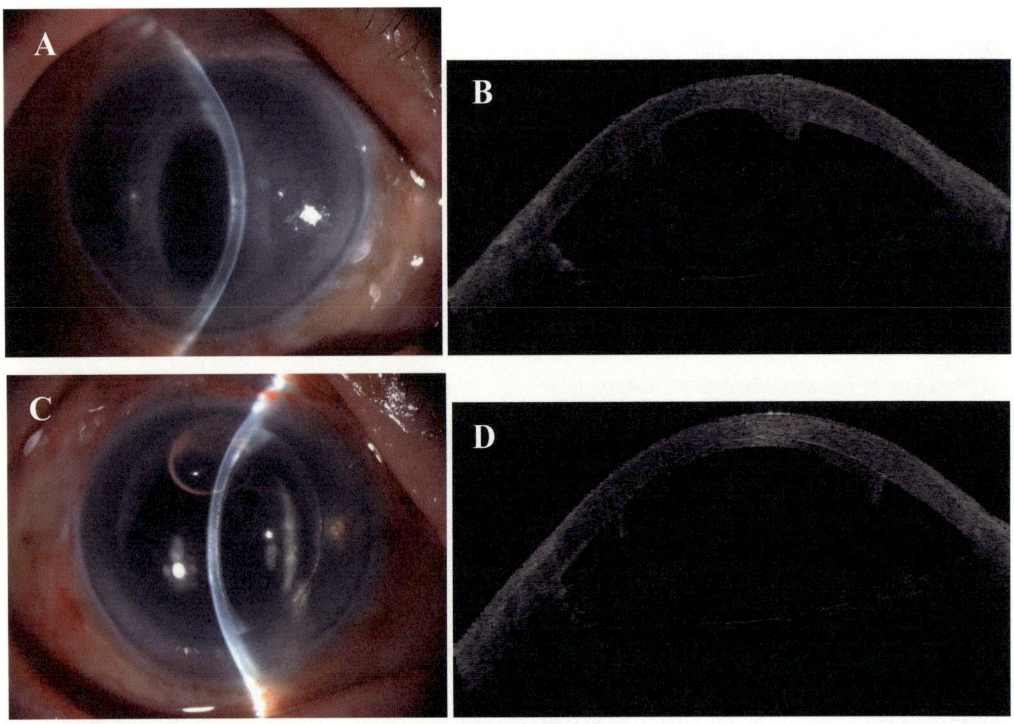

Fig. 3. (case 3) Slit lamp photograph (A) and AS-OCT (B) shows the donor tissue shrink during the first postoperative week. (C) and (D) shows the newly exchanged donor disc is well attached.

3. Discussion

Most manipulations during the DSAEK surgery are performed in the anterior chamber. In addition, at the end of the surgery, air bubble is introduced into the anterior chamber to support the donor graft. Therefore, the stability of the anterior chamber is a critical factor in DSAEK. The natural iris-lens diaphragm is a barrier separating the anterior chamber from posterior vitreous cavity. Patients with anatomically or functionally anomalous iris-lens diaphragm are challenges to DSAEK. Small case series of DSAEK/DSEK were reported in patients with intraoperative floppy-iris syndrome, aphakic patients and aniridic aphakic patients.[1,2,3] The results were largely favorable with some modification of the surgical technique. Bradley et al. described a suture-drag technique to minimize intraoperative donor endothelial trauma in patients with intraoperative floppy-iris syndrome.[1] Price et al. used anchor suture securing the donor to the recipient to prevent the donor tissue from dropping down to the retina in aniridic aphakic eyes.[2] However, since the main purpose of DSAEK is to improve vision, we think it should be more appropriate to correct aphakia and aniridia either prior to or at the same time with DSAEK surgery. Aniridic aphakic patients would benefit from BDI lens that could in some extent compensate optically the loss of iris and crystal lens. However, the BDI lens is not an ideal barrier to maintain a stable anterior chamber compared with the natural iris-lens diaphragm. There is gap between the haptics and the black diaphragm, especially in the traumatic cases without capsular remnants. Therefore, after a 5mm incision was made in DSAEK, the pressure in the anterior chamber will decrease, thus it is unavoidable that the liquefied vitreous humor will go through the gap into the anterior chamber and the pressure of the posterior segment will decline. Anterior irrigation during graft insertion is not enough to compensate this occult vitrous loss. In the presence of pressure difference between the anterior and posterior segment, when the air bubble was injected into the anterior chamber, it would easily go back to the vitreous cavity postoperatively just like what we observed in case 1 in which the graft was found partially detached and the air bubble was totally disappeared on the first postoperative day. Therefore, when DSAEK is considered in an aniridic patient with BDI lens, we recommend that the pressure difference should be balanced first before the donor was unfolded by the air bubble.

Glaucoma is a common complication for both traumatic and congenital aniridia. In the traumatic eye, the trabecular meshwork could easily be jeopardized in the presence of extensive loss of iris tissue. Likewise, anomalous development of the anterior chamber angle in congenital aniridia could result in progressive IOP elevation.[4] In addition, the prevalence of glaucoma will further increased after BDI lens implantation.[5,6] It was ascribed to the continuous irritation of the haptics and the diaphragm to the uveal remnants in congenital aniridia, which may alter the blood–aqueous barrier, accelerating glaucoma progression.[5] It was also proposed that the large size of the BDI lens may impair aqueous outflow by direct compression on the anterior chamber angle.[6] In some cases the haptics of the lens were found not rest in the ciliary sulcus but in the anterior chamber angle.[5] Therefore, use of type 67G BDI lens with smaller haptic diameter (12.5mm) was recommend.[6] Glaucoma was observed in two of our patients (case 1 and case 2) before DSAEK, but could be controlled medically. During the postoperative follow-up, case 1 had a temporary IOP rise, and case 2 experienced a persistent hypertony that was successfully treated with cyclophotocoagulation. In our case series, all three patients were implanted with 67G BDI lens, and the UBM prior to DSAEK surgery showed the haptics of the lens were not in contact with the trabecular meshwork. Therefore, we think angle compression by the haptics is not a major cause for IOP elevation in our cases. However, we do believe that glaucoma is an issue that deserves special attention when DSAEK is planned to be undertaken in aniridic cases with BDI lens. A well control of IOP preoperatively and close postoperative follow-up to monitor the IOP is recommended.

It is also essential to find out the main reasons for endothelial decompensation in these three cases. Trauma can cause endothelial loss. Congenital aniridia could also associate with endothelial deficiency, although the most common corneal change is limbal stem cell deficiency.[7,8] Normally, the BDI lens was sutured to the ciliary sulcus, it should has no friction with the endothelium unless the BDI lens is decentered or displaced anteriorly.[5,6] In our three patients, UBM showed that the BDI lens were in the right position, and the endothelial cell counts before BDI lens implantation were already lower than the normal value. We think that BDI lens did not contribute to endothelial cell loss in our three cases, and thus it was not necessary to remove the lens during DSAEK.

4. References

[1] Bradley JC, McCartney DL. Descemet's stripping automated endothelial keratoplasty in intraoperative floppy-iris syndrome: Suture-drag technique. J Cataract Refract Surg. 2007;33:1149-50.

[2] Price MO, Price FW Jr, Trespalacios R. Endothelial keratoplasty technique for aniridic aphakic eyes. J Cataract Refract Surg. 2007;33:376-9.

[3] Suh LH, Kymionis G, Culbertson WW, et al. Descemet's stripping with endothelial keratoplasty in aphakic eyes. Arch Ophthalmol 2008;126:268 –70.

[4] Grant WM, Walton DS. Progressive changes in the angle in congenital aniridia, with development of glaucoma. Trans Am Ophthalmol Soc. 1974;72:207-28.

[5] Reinhard T, Engelhardt S, Sundmacher R. Black diaphragm aniridia intraocular lens for congenital aniridia: Long-term follow-up. J Cataract Refract Surg. 2000;26:375-81.

[6] Implantation of the Black Diaphragm Intraocular Lens in Congenital and Traumatic Aniridia. Ophthalmology 2008;115:1705–1712

[7] Mackman G, Brightbill FS, Optiz JM. Corneal changes in aniridia. Am J Ophthalmol 1979;87:497–502.

[8] Ramaesh K, Ramaesh T, Dutton GN, Dhillon B. Evolving concepts on the pathogenic mechanisms of aniridia related keratopathy. Int J Biochem Cell Biol. 2005;37:547-57.

Part 3

Complications of Keratoplasties

7

The Complications After Keratoplasty

Patricia Durán Ospina
Fundación Universitaria del Área Andina Seccional Pereira
Colombia

1. Introduction

Keratoplasty is the medical term that refers to a cornea transplant. There are some differences between the definitions of keratoplasty, commonly it is mentioned for corneal transplant, Lamellar Keratoplasty, which is a partial thickness corneal grafting and penetrating keratoplasty: is a full-thickness corneal grafting. The indications for keratoplasty include: optical (to improve visual acuity by replacing the opaque host tissue by a healthy donor or pesudophakic bullous keratopathy), tectonic (in patients with stromal thinning and descemetoceles, to preserves corneal anatomy ant integrity), therapeutic (removal of inflamed corneal tissue refractive to treatment by antibiotics or antiviral drugs) or cosmetic (in patients with corneal scars giving a whitish opaque hue to the cornea.

The most frequent causes of corneal alterations leading to keratoplasty are keratoconus, bacterial infections, poor hygienic contact lens wear (Buehler et al. 1992, Chalupa, 1987, Holden, 2003) or trauma. Among microbial infections, bacterial infections are the most frequent and are mainly caused by *Staphylococcus sp., Streptococcus sp. or Pseudomona sp.*

Some side effects of keratoplasty can be infection (keratitis on the new transplanted cornea or endophthalmitis), transplant rejection, vision fluctuation, glaucoma and bleeding, among others less reported. Infection is one of the most frequent complications after keratoplasty, which can cause endophthalmitis. Infection after keratoplasty, can result from inapropiate healing or like a complication during the transplant (Confino and Brown, 1985 and Dana, 1995). even though the area around the eye is completely sterilized the day of the surgery and the face is covered with sterile drapes. Despite these actions to keep the surgical area clean, infections still may occur.

On the other hand, transplant rejection is one of the hardest complications after keratoplasty. It occurs when the body rejects the new cornea. But it can occur from days to several years after surgery. Symptoms that show that the immunological system has rejected the cornea may be redness of the eye, an extreme sensitivity to light and pain, autoimmune diseases, infiltrates and also unknown causes. Signs of rejection may occur anywhere from one month to several years after the transplant surgery. On these cases, keratoplasty can be repeated when the transplant is rejected and oral immunosupresor drugs must be taken for long time to reduce the rejection. Some authors are reported also vision fluctuation after keratoplasty, frequent symptoms are poor vision and fluctuations for up to several months or years. Not until the vision has reached a constant and the sutures have been removed can the individual be given a prescription for eyeglasses or special contact lenses.

Other reports refer to glaucoma like a potential complication after keratoplasty. Glaucoma is a buildup of pressure in the eye that can cause a complete loss of vision. Keratoplasty increases the chances of pressure buildup during the surgical procedure that may lead to glaucoma for metabolism changes on the stroma or perhaps can be caused for immunological reactions or metabolic associations. It depends of the clinical history of each patient, not all cases are the same, by this reason must be studied independently. Additionally, may appear bleeding and pain after keratoplasty, sometimes the blood vessels may leak, which would result in bleeding from the eyes. In these cases, sitting upright will encourage the blood to settle. Pain after the keratoplasty is a common side effect oftentimes due to dry eyes. In theory the dry eye contribute with corneal infection, probably due to the opportunistic microbes, which invade the tissue, also is the same with the use of contact lenses for long periods due to hypoxia (low oxygen) (Mertz G. 1980) and to hypercapny (increase of carbon dioxide CO_2). Patients usually feel pain and discomfort when they move the eye at all for weeks after surgery.

Ocular infection occurs mostly in immunosuppressed patients, prior diabetes mellitus, hypertension, hypoadrenalism, taking oral corticosteroids, atopic dermatitis; prolonged use and low hygienic conditions with contact lenses (soft lenses are more frequent than RGP contact lenses) , opportunistic microorganisms which interfered with normal flora, dry eye and a low percentage for contamination of the surgical team. The etiology of keratoplasty in cases of microbial infection has been reported by several authors, as well as the findings on postoperative keratoplasty, one of the main causes is keratoconus and previous corneal graft rejection. The most common microbiological findings correspond to bacteria such as *Staphylococcus sp., Pseudomonas sp., Pneumococcus sp. Serratia marcescens, Streptococcus pneumoniae, Streptococcus viridians, Bacillus* sp., *Corynebacterium sp.* primarily and other microorganisms such as fungi (*Candida sp. Candida glabrata, Aspergillus sp., Fusarium* sp.), among the viruses that are mostly found associated with keratoplasty are the *herpes simple*.

In the reports of eye infection as a complication after keratoplasty, the finding of organisms corresponds in most cases to opportunistic bacteria of the normal ocular flora. In a prospective study conducted in 2004 by a team of researchers in Japan (Wakimasu et al. 2004). They found in a retrospective study among 753 eyes with microbial keratitis after keratoplasty, 14 had bacterial and 13 fungal infections. The time intervals between transplantation and the onset of infection averaged were seven months on average for bacteria and 24 for fungus. In many cases unexpected occasions are to be studied independently and allow further studies regarding the appropriate surgical protocol and the use of antibiotic and steroid therapy to prevent such cases in future.

Even reports of mixed infections are: bacteria-bacteria, fungus or bacteria. Associated with these findings should be taken into account the presence of bacterial endotoxins are another complication of keratoplasty of microbial origin, producing toxic anterior segment syndrome (TASS), which has been attributed to the use of intracamerular antibiotics, reusable cannulas, cleaning the instrumental use of detergents or non-ionized water, among others (Maier et al. 2010). Moreover, the time of onset of infection can vary from weeks to years of development after transplantation. The associated risks are contaminated sutures, persistent epithelial defects. The clinical appearance of TASS is typically characterized by intense early postoperative inflammation of the anterior ocular segment. Sometimes it can be accompanied by fibrin formation, corneal edema, without periocular pain. For diagnosis of this pathology it is important to make routine microbial tests: (culture of microorganisms, mycobacteria, polymer chain reaction (PCR), mycoplasm, Chlamydia, simplex virus, adenovirus and endotoxins (limulus amebiocyte lysata, QCL 1000, Cambrex Bio Science).

Some factors to take into account to protect the cornea in these surgeries are prophylactic antibiotic treatment, asepsis eye with an appropriate antiseptic prior to surgery, postoperative antibiotic treatment, age, nutrition and immunosuppressant of the patient and to be taken considered minimizing the risk of postsurgical infection. Before this surgical procedure should be performed before the control protocol for signs or symptoms of eye infection and make an effective and timely microbiologic diagnosis. In the case of mixed microbial infections reported leading to keratoplasty (bacteria-bacteria or bacteria-fungi) (Garcia et al.2004, Delgado et al.2008), it should be clear which is the microorganism more dangerous to invade cornea (fungus or bacteria) to inhibit it with the indicated treatment (antimycotic or antibiotic agent, respectively) , knowing the physiopathology of the infection, the mechanisms of adhesion (biofilm formed for bacteria or hyphaes for fungus) and reflect on the use of corticosteroids in ocular infection, because it which may exacerbate the corneal infection in most cases with corneal compromise. Asepsis previous eye surgery, irrigating with povidone-iodine a day before surgery, has proved a good choice to prevent infection after the keratoplasty (Nash et al. 1991).

Corneal complications due to other ophthalmic surgeries like post intraocular implants relation have been associated with edema. It occurs for many reasons, but it is often a sequel of intraocular surgery, called either pseudophakic bullous keratopathy (PBK) or aphakic bullous keratopathy (ABK). Knowledge of the structure of the cornea and the proper functioning of its layers is fundamental to understanding corneal edema. Authors suggest that the endothelium becomes increasingly unable to act as a pump to deturgesce the cornea, it causes the stroma begins to swell, especially in the central cornea. As the stroma swells, the cornea thickens and folds are seen in the Descemet membrane. The edema may fluctuate in response to changing intraocular pressure with higher pressures leading to more edema. At this point, maintenance of intraocular pressure at a low level is important. The combination of variable endothelial function and variable intraocular pressure determines the extent of corneal edema (Aquavella et al, 2010).

This chapter is a description of microbial complications in keratoplasty, to understand the physiology and behavior of these microorganisms in the surgical process, the relationship with the ocular immune system at the time of surgery, knowing the clinical findings to identify whether a bacterial infection, viral or fungal infection may be present. Another factor to evaluate the postoperative course of keratoplasty is the type of antibiotic used after keratoplasty and should be evaluated according to clinical evidence, since in many cases is not time for microbiological culture fungal or bacterial infection alone is assessed, but fungi attack the corneal stroma, being more aggressive with corneal tissues:

Microbial complications post-keratoplasty may even become worse on endophthalmitis and in the worst cases enucleating of some inevitable cases. In vitro studies, it have shown that the anatomy of corneal tissue which allows the invasion of microorganisms in and its biochemical composition. The corneal stroma lamellar structure composed of collagen fibrils which contribute to corneal transparency, being invaded by microorganisms allows rapid entry stromal inflammatory cells, predisposing to ulcers. Crystalline keratopathy caused by *Streptococcus sp*. should not confuse with a fungal infection because it form a crystalline forms similar to mycotic hyphaes. (Butler et al.2001).

2. Statistical methods

2.1 Method

For the analysis of the data, the following sources were consulted for this paper: Expert opinion, clinical case reports and specialized databases. In the first case, it was a survey with ophthalmologists skilled in corneal surgery, yielding six National specialists which are located geographically in Colombia. An unstructured interview was used for this. For the clinical reports, we reviewed the clinical cases of the service of ophthalmic consult of Fundación Universitaria del Área Andina Seccional Pereira and the reports made by specialists.

2.2 Databases

Three bibliographic databases were searched: Medline, Ebsco, Hinary. To facilitate the search, the connector used was "and". In total 78 Articles were reviewed and 37 were chosen for the report.

2.3 Keywords

Keratoplasty,ophthalmology, ocular and immunology, keratoplasty and complications, microbiological infections and cornea.

2.4 Criteria for inclusion

First, personal meeting with experts (ophthalmologist cornea specialists) was conducted for the review. Second, we reviewed clinical cases of the optometric clinical of Fundación Universitaria del Area Andina Seccional Pereira and private ophthalmologist consult. Additionally, the inclusion criteria respond to the search of articles and reports of work based on post keratoplasty infection, immunological and post-keratoplasty complications, astigmatism and post-keratoplasty using End Notes. The clinical cases selection was made by ophthalmological consult of control with complications post-keratoplasty. Three cases were included.

2.5 Criteria for exclusion

Articles with the topic of ocular infections which did not require keratoplasty, and immunological diseases without corneal compromises, were rejected.

3. Clinical pearls on microbial complications after and before keratoplasty

The most microbial reported associated with microbial keratitis which required keratoplasty are bacterial associations (Driebe and Stern 1983) following by mycotic and herpetic infections and less often, *Acanthamoeba sp*. The complications are more dangerous if there is an association with corneal stroma because the cornea needs respiration (Hill, 1976). Several factors contribute to adherence (Miller,1987) by bacteria: extracellular bacterial products such as alkaline proteases, protease IV, exotoxin A, exo-enzyme B and a recent small protease, called PASP (*P. aeruginosa* small protease) are been reported and contributes to epithelial erosions in keratitis caused by this agent. Recently, a group of molecules bacterial signaling, known as N-acilhomoserina lactones (AHLs), has also been reported as important factors in virulence of same bacterias (Marquart et al., 2005). The correlation between these factors of adherence and virulence, as the production of signals of molecular and expression of phenotypic characteristics including the production of enzymes, has studied by chromatography and bioassay in recent years. Moreover, the lack of tear that low lubrication caused by widespread use is a factor that should be taken into account users contact lenses (Kwong, 2007), because the tear is carrier lysozyme, lactoferrin, and immunoglobulins ®-lysine that being dehydrated lens facilitates molecular adhesion of *P. aeruginosa* (Zhu et al. 2002).

3.1 Differential diagnosis between keratitis caused by microbes

There are a lot of reason for make microbial culture collection in all protocols to identify the type of microbial keratitis pre or post keratoplasty: Signs are similar in bacterial keratitis, exist mixed infections which required different treatments, there are several signs can help to make the differential diagnosis prior to the results of the microbiological findings, some of these are:

SIGNS	BACTERIAL KERATITIS	MYCOTIC KERATITIS	HERPES KERATITIS	ACANTHAMOEBA KERATITIS
Hyperemy	Yes	Yes	Yes	Yes
Satellite lesion	No	Yes	No	No
Pain	Yes	Yes	Yes (Active lession)	Yes
Lession borders	Regular	Diffused and irregulars, Feathery borders or hyphate edges	Dendritic ulcers	Regular
Hypopyon	Yes or no	which appears dry, rough, and leathery	No	No
Color infiltrates	White, cream, yellow	infiltrates appear grayish-white or yellowish-white, and the base of the ulcer is often filled with soft, creamy, raised exudates, dematiaceousfungi: brown or black pigmentation on the surface of the ulcer.	White	White or grey
Frequent Causes	corneal foreign body, contact with non-sterile water, bullous keratopathy, neurotrophic keratopathy, herpes simplex keratitis, radial keratotomy, swimming and scuba diving, basement membrane dystrophy, contact lens wear and bacterial keratitis	Vegetal origin foreign body contamination, dirty case lenses storage, immunosupression.	Immuno-supression	Contaminated water, dirty contact lens case contaminated
Micro-organisms	*Staphylococcus sp., Streptococcus sp., Pseudomona sp.Mycobacterium sp.*	*Aspergillus sp, Fusarium sp., Candida sp.* (Muzaliha et al.,2010)	*Herpes simple*	*Acanthamoeba sp.* (McCulley,2000) (Varga et al.1993)
Stromal immunological ring	No	No	No	Immunological ring at the limbus

Table 1. Microbes finding on clinical pearls of keratitis complications associated with corneal infections after keratoplasty and common treatment.

Some infections are caused by more than one microorganism of different species, some of the normal flora or anothers opportunistic microbes like different bacteria species and in even and rare cases fungi and bacteria. It has been reported more frequently in contact lens wearers in widespread use without improper lubrication, as in the case of Figure 1, a case reported by our research group, where the patient also had a cosmetic tattoo in her eyes. On these cases perhaps an alteration of the normal flora associated with corneal dehydration can contribute to the eye injury. Some cases of contamination should be detected early and obligatorily required to perform a microbial culture using PCR techniques to detect it in less time and be very cautious with antibiotic and steroid therapy in these special patients. Steroids may get worse the damage still unknown causes andantibacterial antibiotics do not work against fungi. The review of these protocols and prior detection signs is the key to the success of a good corneal transplant.

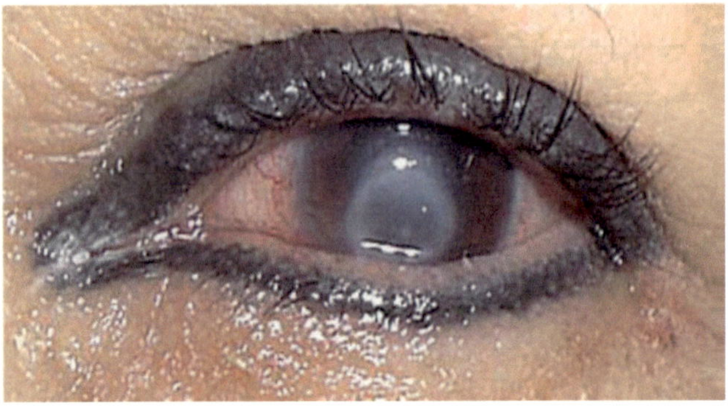

Fig. 1. Infection before keratoplasty caused by Mixed flora: Bacterial keratitis and *Aspergillus sp.*, six days evolution. (Delgado, Chile. 2008, Photograph Personal Album: Márquez & Durán).

In the microbial ocular infections, those with bacterial association respond in most cases if the lesson is peripherical, if the lesson is central and affects optical zone, are more likely to result finally in keratoplasty, perhaps the periphery limbal vessels contribute to improved immune performance, while in central corneal recovery is slower and microbial invasion penetrates more easily to the stroma. But in the case of fungal infections, those fungal cases are caused in most cases for vegetal origin, inappropriately use of contact lenses or unknown causes. In China, in a study performed from 2000 to 2008 with 899 patients, they found no recovery when the treatment was made combined conjunctiva or intracamerular fluconazol. (Shi et. al. 2010). By the other hand, therapy with silver sulfadiazine ointment, natamycin is a better prognosis in cases of microbial infections of fungal origin. Another authors include cyclosporine to prevent graft rejection beginning 2 weeks after penetrating keratoplasty (PKP) and avoid steroids (Xie et al., 2001). Steroids for unknown cause in the case of fungus and bacteria like *Pseudomona* are not a good choice for treatment and cannot be administrated for the security of the corneal integrity. More studies are required in a future for new options of immunossupressor against immunological mediator of inflammation. It is important to check any graft rejection, clarity of the graft, visual acuity, and surgical complications after surgery in all cases.

3.2 Treatment of microbial infections after keratoplasty

The successful treatment of microbial infections requires of the experience of an interdisciplinary team: corneal experts ophthalmologists, immunologists and microbiologists

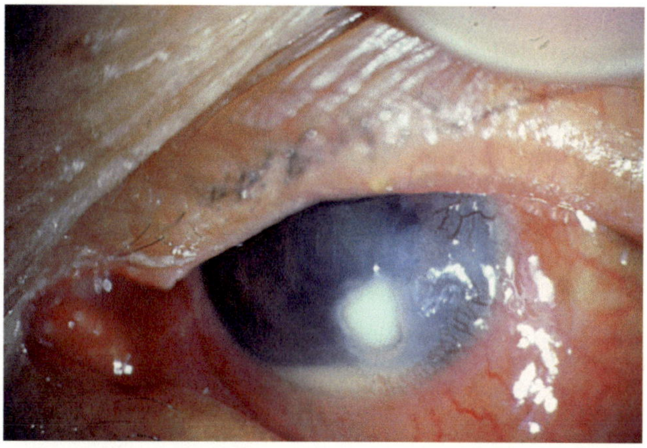

Fig. 2. Keratitis and posterior endophtalmitis infection caused by *Staphylococcus sp.* (Courtesy: Ophthalmologist Emilio Méndez.M.D. Personal Atlas).

and the cooperation of the patient. It is important to act fast and certainly. The use of antibiotics like last generation fluoroquinolones is the best option and it is recognized around the world in the case of bacterial complications. With the fungus infections it is not easy, due that it is hard to have the microbiological findings on time. For these reason the clinical pearls are so important to choice the best therapy.
These are the antibiotic therapies recommended for experts:

MICROORGANISMS	ANTIBIOTICS FOR TREATMENT	ANTIMICOTICS AGENTS
Staphylococcus sp. *Streptococcus sp.*	Vancomicine, Moxifloxacine, Ciprofloxacine	No
Mycobacterium sp.	Amikacin,cefoxitin, clarithromycin	No
Fusarium sp.	No	Amphotericin B or Natamycin or silver sulfadiazine, intrastomal variconazole.
Fusarium sp. +*Pseudomona sp.*	Ciprofloxacin, Moxifloxacine, Gatifloxacine, Vancomicine (against *Pseudomona sp.*)	Amphotericin B or Natamycin or silver sulfadiazine (against *Fusarium sp.*), intrastomal variconazole.
Candida sp.	No	Amphotericin B or Natamycin or silver sulfadiazine, intrastomal variconazole.

Table 2. Microbes finding on keratitis complications associated with corneal infections after keratoplasty and common treatment.

In the case of infection caused by *Acanthamoeba sp.,* propamidine isethionate 0.1% ophthalmic solution administrated concomitantly with neomycin-polymyxin B gramicidin ophthalmic solution has shown best results. Against neovascularization, another therapy has been used, topical bevacizumab, a humanized monoclonal antibody that recognizes and blocks vascular endothelial growth factor A (VEGF-A). VEGF-A is a chemical signal that stimulates the growth of new blood vessels (angiogenesis) in graft rejection (Saxena, 2009). The scientists reported successfully results in one case of graft rejection 6 months following penetrating keratoplasty (triple procedure) in the left eye. With the administration of topical bevacizumab (4 mg/4 mL) in a dose of one drop twice a day for 15 days, she improved her vision and this short topical bevacizumab therapy, may potentially offer a safer and more effective alternative in treating graft rejection after penetrating keratoplasty. The administration must be subconjunctival also, and it is in study for side effects.

3.3 Immunological findings after keratoplasty

One of the major complications associated with corneal graft rejection post-keratoplasty associations are immune from the donor and recipient. The therapy with immunomodulators before and after treatment required an individual protocol like a great option to prevent such rejection. Corneal transplantation is a continuous release of antigens in the different corneal layers of specific immune response against the donor cornea. This rejection may occur soon after surgery or month and years later. The following table specifies the associated warning signs in case of rejection and to be taken into account in the post-operative:

Studies in animal models (mice) based on corneal transplantation have shown that the main mediators of the immune response implicated in cases of graft rejection are CD4 cells Th1, Th2, CD4+, CD25+ and recently and hypothesis that Th17 play a crucial role in allograft rejection (Cunnusamy, 2010). Also, eosinophils secrete an array of cytotoxic granule cationic proteins such as major basic protein (MBP), eosinophil cationic protein (ECP), eosinophile peroxidase (EPO), eosinophil-derived neurotoxin (EDN) which are capable of inducing tissue damage and dysfunction (Gleich et al, 1993) and after this findings new chemical mediators are involved in this toxicity like eotaxin, a chemokine that attracts eosinophils to bind to its specific receptor, could induce the proliferation of fibroblasts, leading to the excretion of collagen. Fibroblasts also secrete eotaxin when stimulated by IL-4 and tumor necrosis factor (TNF) (Kumagai et al, 2005). Additionally, one might think in the research based on inhibition of those toxins for therapy pre and post-keratoplasty in a future to minimize their toxic effects, which ones contribute to graft rejection. Some like the studies on mices in recent years, which are trying to use IFN-γ for inhibit eotaxin expression at both: protein and mRNA levels, in cultured human corneal fibroblasts. This effect of IFN-γ may contribute to the inhibition of eosinophil infiltration into the cornea. Exogenous IFN-γ thus represents a potential new therapeutic agent for the treatment of corneal disorders associated with inflammatory ocular diseases such as vernal keratoconjunctivitis.(Fukuda et al. 2002). Some patients present immunological events of rejection after years of POP, perhaps to systemic immunological complications that must be studied in each case with immunological analysis.

TYPE OF FAILURE OF THE IMPLANT	PRIMARY FAILURE	LATE FAILURE
Time of occurrence	Graft failure after first days of postoperatory	Graft failure after months or years after postoperatory
Signs	Edema after surgery, low transparency during the firsts weeks	Gradual diffuse edema, increase corneal infiltrates, corneal vascularization

Epithelial failure	Occurs in two forms that respond to steroid use. The patient is asymptomatic or has minimal skin irritation. It is self-limiting and does not change in the visual acuity (V.A.). • The first type is characterized by elevated epithelial rejection line that stains with fluorescein or rose bengal. Progresses rapidly in days to 2 weeks and may take the form of a ring concentric to the limbus, peripheral to the interface area and subsequently shrinks to the center. The line represents an area of destruction of donor epithelium, which is covered by host epithelium. • The second type is characterized by the presence of subepithelial infiltrates, which contain lymphocytes. They are similar in appearance to those produced by adenovirus. Can change shape, location and disappear by themselves.
Stromal failure	It is accompanied usually of endothelial rejection. It is characterized by a haze peripheral full-thickness, limbal injection in a previously clear corneal button. Infiltration can be identified in the peripheral interface progresses centrally
Endothelial failure	A classic rejection presents with endothelial rejection line (Khodadoust, 2008), which usually begins in a vascularized portion of the interface and progresses, if untreated, through the endothelial surface over several days. It consists of mononuclear white cells damage the endothelium. This line is made up of mononuclear cells (white blood cells that appear at the vascularized edge of the recently transplanted cornea, if untreated, the line of white blood cells move across and damage the endothelial cells of the cornea. There may be a reaction of moderate to severe CA. The damaged endothelium cannot maintain adequate dehydration of the button and the swells in the posterior to the line, while before it is transparent. Another variant of endothelial rejection presents with diffuse keratic precipitates and anterior chamber reaction, stromal edema localized but not widespread and limbal injection.
Risk factors	Vascularization on the base layers of the recipient corneal. It is the only factor whose relationship to the increased incidence of rejection has been demonstrated. It is believed to be due to loss of immune privilege of the cornea due to normal avascularity
	Large and eccentric grafts
	Incompatibility of HLA-A, HLA-B and ABO group
	History of previous rejection of any kind
	Bilateral Keratoplasty
	Preservation transportation media and corneal tissue pre - transplantation
	Age
	Presence of epithelium in a donor transplant
	Association with atopic dermatitis, allergy and asthma

Table 3. Types of corneal transplant failure

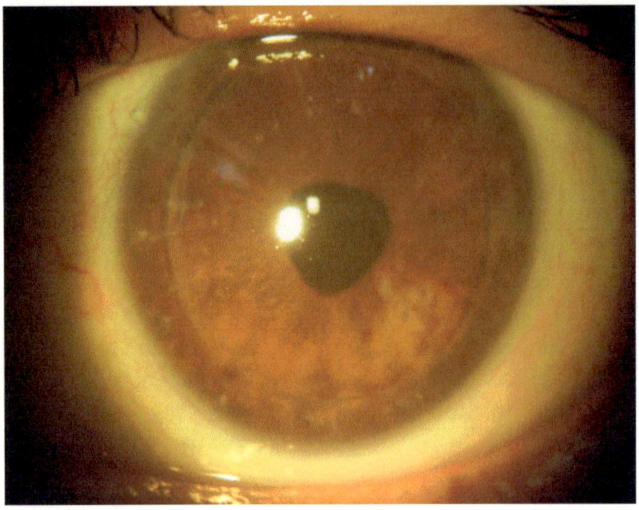

Fig. 3. Keratitis infiltrates post-keratoplasty after 13 year of postoperatory of the keratoplasty. (Cortesy: Mayra Cáceres O.D.)

Another chemical mediator of immune response (Awadi, 2011) are metalloproteinases, collagenase, stomelysin and gelatinase. These matrix of metalloproteinases are inhibited by specific endogenous tissue inhibitors of metalloproteinases (TIMP1, TIMP2, TIMP3, TIMP4), like batimastat and marimastat. Modulation of metalloproteinase activity may thus help to model and minimize scarring such as that occurring in ketatoconus or after traumatic or surgical injury to the cornea (See Chapter Modeling of corneal healing and corneal inflammatory response). Those findings will be so useful to performer better protocols for receptors and immunological exam before and after surgery.

Recent research on bovine serum- free corneal cell and wounded organ cultures were developed with a range of concentrations of TGF- TGF-β1, -β2, and -β3; IL-10; and neutralizing human monoclonal antibodies (mAbs) against TGF-β1 in order to watch the inhibition of TGF-β for reduce the myofibroblast differentiation and fibrosis in the cornea, this results may contribute in a future to determined the actions of distinct TGF-β isoforms and their inhibitors during early corneal wound healing is an essential step in guiding therapeutic intervention. The found that TGF- β1 delayed re-epithelization, increased repopulation of the stroma, increase proliferation and was the only isoform to promote myofibroblast differentiation. Aditionally, IL-10 promoted corneal re-epithelialization at low doses but inhibited this response at high doses. Stromal repopulation was prevented by all doses of IL-10. TGF-β2 or the anti-TGF-β2 mAb, CAT-152 had little effect on any repair parameter. Treatment with the anti-TGF-β1 accelerates corneal re-epithelialization but reduces cell repopulation of the stroma. The cytokines TGF-β3 and IL-10 have opposing actions to that of TGF-β1. (Carrington L. et al. 2006).

By the other hand, the evolution of new surgical techniques have been improving for keratoplasty, as well as treatment protocols and prevention of graft rejection, beginning with the removal of sutures to secure the graft, in 1956, using a posterior approach, first reported for Tillett, in 1998, Dr. Gerritt Melles et al. described posterior lamellar keratoplasty (PLK) technique that uses air instead of sutures, placement of the graft to the recipient cornea. Their technique required initial lamellar dissection of the donor and recipient cornea, excision of a 7.5 mm diameter recipient posterior stroma 7.0 button with attached endothelium and the insertion of a posterior donor button size similar through a limbal incision mm-9. Later, Melles et al. then doubled the donor graft that could be inserted through an incision of 5 mm. Another technique used to simplify the procedure was published by Dr. Goroyov, using a microkeratome to harvest the donor graft, a variation known as Descemet's endothelial keratoplasty automated extraction (DSAEK). Besides reducing the technical difficulty of the general procedure, descemetorhexis and microkeratome donor dissection was also softer surface receptor and donor, resulting in more satisfactory visual results. In 2006, Melles al. et al reported a success with a new variant called Descemet membrane endothelial keratoplasty (DMEK) involved in transplanting endothelium naked DM - a specific disease true form of keratoplasty with minimal trauma.

In 2008, Dr. Pavel Studeny showed a variation of this technique at the American Academy of Ophthalmology annual meeting 2008, which formed a "huge bubble" of air to separate the center of 6 mm or less of the donor, separating the posterior stroma by manual lamellar dissection, removed the stroma during the great bubble and marked central tissue from a donor with the appropriate diameter to create a graft that was naked and central DM endothelium with stroma attached outer edge. This configuration allows easier handling and graft insertion or DSAEK/DMEK anyone. He recently had a variation of this technique called automated keratoplasty endothelial Descemet membrane (DMAEK), in which the donor tissue is first dissected with a microkeratome as DSAEK, a large central bubble is formed, the overlying stroma is removed large bubble, and the fabric is pierced with a drill. All those surgical techniques among others, contribute to reduce the inflammatory response by chemical mediators of inflammation reducing the reject of the implant and are so important for future immunological research and found a long term protocol and also epidemiological studies between those techniques and the relationship with the receptor immunological reject. But it must take in mind each patient's medical history, previous history of atopic dermatitis, systemic and ocular allergies, several dry eye and systemic associations such as diabetes, hypertension and especially those of an autoimmune rheumatoid arthritis, atopic dermatitis, among others to make a very good rating diagnosis before graft itself to the corneal donor. New alternatives based on artificial biopolymers are been introduced in recent researches, and it is mainly important to study the biocompatibility and immune response of these new technologies with the human ocular tissue.

Another new technique to performance keratoplasty is the femtosecond Laser-Assisted Lamellar Keratoplasty, which reduce intraoperative complications, additionally, optimizes postoperative refraction, allows faster visual rehabilitation, and decreases the risk of graft rejection and astigmatism, this technique permits create vertical and lamellar corneal incisions with a variety of shapes and angulations at a precise depth. Combining the advantages of lamellar keratoplasty with the surgical precision of a femtosecond laser enables us new surgical options. Femtosecond laser-assisted lamellar keratoplasty techniques include femtosecond laser-assisted anterior lamellar keratoplasty (FALK), femtosecond laser-assisted deep anterior lamellar keratoplasty (FDALK), and femtosecond laser-assisted endothelial keratoplasty (FLEK), (Yoo,S,Hurmeric V, 2011). The authors recommend performed in patients with deep stromal scarring, keratoconus and ectasia.

Recent research led by scientists from Stanford University with a technique called advance Dolhman-Doane, which consists of a core of plastic biopolymer, transparent and tough, which is surrounded with human tissue and could be an alternative in countries where the corneal donation is not as accequible. For attachment to the rest of the globe, further chemical engineer Curtis Frank has created an artificial cornea polyacrylic acid and polyethylene nets, achieving a transparent material with high water content 80%. Future research is needed to view and evaluate the biocompatibility in vivo metabolic behavior with other nutrients to the cornea and allow epithelial cells attaching to the surface to prevent risk of infection acting as a layer of protection. Additionally, the bioengineer Jennifer Cochran came up with the addition of collagen to a surface of artificial cornea for better grip and other scientific using the technique of photolithography (manufacture of semiconductor materials) Frank and his team can also create patterns of microscopic pores around the edge of the implant. Thus, when the cornea is implanted in her patient's eye, the cells migrated through the pores by anchoring the cornea in the eye and helping to integrate the artificial material with natural tissue. This process reduces the number of sutures necessary to maintain the artificial cornea into place (Technology Review, MIT). There are major projects being carried out to sensitize the artificial cornea implants as the CORNEA EU project to produce artificial cornea has prompted efforts Joachim Storsberg, the Fraunhofer Institute for Applied Polymer Research IAP in German. His work has led to the creation of new versions of the artificial cornea implants has been shown to have less risk in terms of eye injuries.

3.4 Another risk factors of post-keratoplasty complications

Despite of microbiological and immunological complications are significant to prevent rejection. Those are relationship with the age of the receptor. The allograft rejection has been reported more common in children than in adults, possibly due to a more active immune system in younger patients. On those patients the pediatric transplant sometimes not without clear evidence of endothelial rejection. The rejection may even many years after transplantation. If irreversible failure occurs in patients in the age range amblyogenic, regrafting still may be indicated to advance the patient's visual development. Glaucoma is another common complication on these patients; also ocular hypertension can damage the optic nerve and threaten the survival of the graft and therefore the visual prognosis. The vulnerability of glaucoma in pediatric keratoplasty is potentially affected by the anterior segment abnormal structure or the use of steroids after surgery. Other complications, including endophthalmitis, choroidal hemorrhage, cataract, retinal detachment and phthisis bulbi are relatively rare but do occur.

Another authors reported Suture-related graft infection is a serious complication after penetrating keratoplasty and often leads to serious visual lost attributable to scarring, allograft reactions and also increased astigmatism. To reduce the risk of infection, they propose that it is necessary to ensure at each visit all sutures, that knots are well buried and that the sutures are covered by epithelium (Sonavane A. et al, 2003).

In the case of penetrating keratoplasty, the secondary astigmatism post penetrate keratoplasty (PK) is another complication to consider when using this technique. The first factors that may influence the refractive outcome is PK preexisting pathology in the recipient cornea, such as keratoconus, trauma and other causes of thinning or irregularity, especially peripheral, and therefore persist in the transplanted cornea. In cases of keratoconus, astigmatism may see a gradual change over the years, after an initial refractive result QP correct, due to thinning and corneal ecstasy ring at the receiver. Due to scarring, vascularization, the degrees of tension may form irregularities. Additionally, systemic diseases such as diabetes, collagen disease, recipient age, may also affect healing. The more homogeneous it is smaller the astigmatic error. During surgery, there are other parameters

to take into account to prevent complications: compression or deformation of the globe, ocular tone down a narrow cleft interpalpebral a misplaced speculum, a thread tension of the upper rectum or scleral support ring misplaced which can distort the cornea during the trephination and cause a receiver window oval or distorted.
During surgery it is necessary to have a team that includes appropriate microsurgical instruments apart from the ideal, a proper system illumination and a keratoscope surgical microscope. Postoperatively, many factors can also influence the final astigmatism, age, existing disease into the receiver, local and systemic steroid use local time each suture is kept before being withdrawn, leaving them to favor reports longer. It should be up on the controls to show signs of possible rejection, early withdrawal of sutures, traumatic or spontaneous ectasia, epithelial problems, and secondary infection. We must decide, first, the diameter of the graft and the window. Often it will be a compromise between including all opaque or affected area on one side and try not to reach the peripheral vascularized limb or other areas in order to minimize the risk of rejection.
The suture is probably the main factor that may influence the prevention or induction of astigmatism QP. It is important to correctly position each and every one of the points because one of them misplaced can induce astigmatism may not be discovered until the sutures are removed and can be difficult to correct with a secondary procedure. 10-0 nylon monofilament is still the reference material for the final suture button, but in reality is biodegradable and often breaks into a period of one to three years. The 10-0 polypropylene (Prolene) looks like a really material unchanged, but noted that eventually loses its tensile strength and cracked by the action of UV rays. Polyester (like Dacron, Mersilene) is a truly non-resorbable material, and thickness of 11-0 has a similar strength to nylon 10-0. It is a little less elastic and therefore requires a closer fit with the help of keratoscope (the Mersilene of 10-0 should not be used, it is much rigid). Its hydrophobic behavior also avoids the tendency of nylon to join the cause and viscoelastic "soap films." The mersilene 11-0 is another good choice (Barraquer at al. 2002).

4. Time of rejection of the corneal implant

According to the evidence of rejection time after surgery the rejection must be classified in hyperacute, acute or chronic rejection. The hyperacute rejection occurs within days after transplantation of the graft. This type of rejection has become rare, affecting less than 1% of transplant recipients due to improved pre-transplant projections. Hyperacute rejection occurs when the host antibodies recognize and bind to antigens of the graft (such as ABO blood group proteins or proteins of major histocompatibility complex). The binding of these antibodies lead to the initiation of the complement cascade, neutrophil recruitment, platelet activation, endothelial cell damage of the graft, and stimulation of coagulation reactions, which in turn lead to rapid thrombosis, loss of vascular integrity, heart tissue, and loss of graft function.
The acute rejection occurs in approximately fifty percent of transplant recipients experience acute rejection (with only 10% progressing to graft loss), which can occur several hours or days (even weeks) after transplantation. The incidence of acute rejection has decreased significantly with the successful use of immunosuppressants such as cyclosporine and azathioprine. The incidence of graft loss was reduced by the latest anti-rejection treatments. Acute rejection occurs when alloantigen-reactive T cells from the host to infiltrate the graft and become activated by contact with foreign proteins, related to the graft presented to

them by antigen presenting cells. These T cells can lead to tissue damage of the graft by the direct elimination of graft cells (killer T cells) or the production of proinflammatory cytokines such as tumor necrosis factor, interleukin-1, and interferon. These cytokines are vasoactive and perpetuate the inflammatory cell recruitment and infiltration. As a result, graft inflammation progresses, leading to tissue distortion, vascular insufficiency, and cell destruction - all of which may eventually compromise graft function.

By the other hand, the chronic rejection occurs in 50% of transplant patients within 10 years after transplantation. This form of rejection is characterized by the development of occlusion of blood vessels luminal progressive thickening of the intima of medium and large artery walls. Chronic rejection is a pathological response of the tissue remodeling that takes place at a variable rate after graft endothelial cells are traumatized by mechanical damage, ischemia, and immune system during and after the transplant. Damaged vascular endothelial cells produce cytokines and tissue growth factors that initiate vascular repair, causing the underlying smooth muscle cells to begin proliferating. Large amounts of intimal matrix occur, leading to vascular wall thickening stop growing. Slowly progressive reduction in blood flow, results in regional tissue ischemia, cell death and tissue fibrosis.

5. Conclusion

Keratoplasty is one of the ocular surgeries that contribute with the reinsertion to job and daily activities and quality life of patients. For these reason, it is very important to study the complications and how to protect cornea before and after keratoplasty for visual health and integrity of the eye and to prevent it. There are new diagnostic techniques so useful worldwide (PCR, new chromogenic agar, immunological test, diagnostic test) to identify the microbes and to choice the good therapy. The reports of the type of microorganisms which cause the lesions are not the same in all countries: In Asia, mycotic infections are most frequent than in America, where bacterial reports of microbial infections are most frequent listed on literature.

Protocols to perform microbial sampling to identify not only bacteria, but also fungi, viruses and acanthamoeba and also immunological test should be a requirement for the protocol clinical management of infection after corneal transplantation, as well as the overall health status of the patient habits and systemic associations to prevent corneal damage. More and more cases appear around the world, by one or other reasons, and it is important to take care of the type of microorganism present, the therapeutic protocol: signs, culture and treatment. New therapeutic drugs must be studied, especially for fungus findings, like variconazole, and take special care for mix infections: bacteria-fungus for the differential diagnosis. Dry eye or not lubrication can contribute to microbial infections, because the tears are the immune protection for the cornea and the artificial tears help to remove toxins and mycotic spores. Some cases needs treatment immediately but the use or corticoids it is not recommended because it can decrease the immune response against the infection. There are no therapy against endotoxins that are responsible of the major damage of the stromal tissue, causing toxic anterior segment syndrome (TASS) and new techniques of therapy like the use of intracamerular antibiotics, and some recommendations like the use of non-ionized water or detergents during surgery must be evaluated to include in protocols. Another factor to have on mind to prevent infections after keratoplasty is the immunological associations with systemic diseases, and also the maintenance of the cleaning regimen for contact lenses. It is main important for next studies to evaluate if the previous permanent make up for esthetical reasons around the eye, perhaps it can interfere the microbial equilibrium of normal flora and let the opportunistic flora to colonize the eye and cause infections. Among some aftercare corneal transplant recommendations after this finding around the world it should look the next factors:

- Integrity of sutures
- Ephitelization
- Prevention of rejection (immunological exams before surgery donor and receptor)
- More research for therapy protocols
- Non-filtration.

To prevent post surgical infections the disinfection protocols are the main factor to consider for minimize complications: before starting the surgical procedures, all of the recipient eyes (including eyelids and conjunctiva) can be rinsed with povidone iodine solution, 5%, that was allowed to act for 3 to 5 minutes. After drying the periocular surface, the operation field was covered with sterile drapes and PK can be performed as follows: rinsed with sterile solution (balanced salt solution, it is recommended to introduce acetylcholine chloride (like Miochol-E) into the anterior chamber. Prior to donor trephination and the graft's sutural fixation, the donor's endothelium was covered by sodium hyaluronate, 1% (Healon ophthalmic viscosurgical device). To fix the grafts, a double-running cross-stitch suture with 10-0. And the use of an antibiotic ointment administered at the end of surgery.

It is important also instruct patients avoid restrictions and talk about postsurgical care to prevent fails. Some of these are: To take de prescription of antibiotics and drugs, and the restriction recommended by American Ophthalmology Association:

1. Use metal shield nightly or when taking a nap during the day and a cloth pad under glasses during the waking day, for 1 month.
2. Not bend at the waist for more than 10 minutes at a time, but may squat at the knees.
3. Not lift or push anything heavier than 15 pounds, including grandchildren, for 2 weeks.
4. Hair may be gently shampooed by a friend or a beauty shop with the head leaning slightly backwards for 2 weeks.
5. May watch TV
6. No heavy exercise of any kind for 3 weeks
7. No sexual intercourse for 3 days after surgery.
8. No swimming for 3 weeks.
9. Not read for more than 10 minutes at a time for 2 weeks.
10. Walking is permitted.

Other important recommendations to verify are:

Recruitment of donor tissue : de donor must be removed within six hour after death, the viable storage period of the removed cornea-scleral button is two weeks, grafts donors < 12 months or > 70 years are preferably not to be used and for more security it is also important not use corneas from death of unknown causes, certain infectious diseases like Jacob-Creutzfeld, SSPE, progressive multifocal, leuko-encephalopathy (CNS), certain systemic infection (AIDS, septicemia, syphilis, viral hepatitis), leukemia and disseminated lymphoma, intrinsic eye diseases (tumors, active inflammations, previous intra-ocular surgery), with respect to the recipient cornea : absence of corneal sensations, stromal vascularization, corneal thinning at the expected recipient-donor margin, active inflammation) and also it is so important to verify the surgical procedure : decide about graft size, usually graft size is no bigger than 8,5 mm in diameter to avoid post-keratoplasty increase in intra-ocular pressure, anterior synechiae and vascularization. An ideal size is 7,5 mm. Smaller sizes would give rise to astigmatism due to subsequent tissue tension. Excision of donor tissue consists of trephining the corneo-scleral button previously excised from the cadaver. Trephination (cutting) is performed with the donor graft endothelial side up in a concave Teflon block. The donor button is to be 0,5 mm larger than the planned recipient opening.

For less complications, it is main important also to verify excision of recipient tissue, the size of pupils (miosed pre-keratoplasty to avoid injuring the lens and causing cataract), the sterilization process for trephination if is manual, motorized, or vacuum trephine, rapid decompression of the eye is to be avoided. Partial thickness cut is hence performed first, than full-thickness trephination is performed. Four cardinal interrupted sutures are applied at 12, 3, 6, and 9 o'clock respectively. Interrupted or running sutures are then performed. The anterior chamber volume is reformed by injecting Balanced Salt Solution (BSS). Another post-keratoplasty care treatment is: the use of topical steroids QID and Mydriatic solution BID instilled in the operated eye for the next four weeks. Topical steroids should be continued QD for 6 months, the QOD for another 6 months. Early complications include flat anterior chamber, persistent epithelial defects, and infection. Late complications include glaucoma, astigmatism, late wound separation, cystoid macular edema, and recurrence of the initial disease in the donor graft. Graft failure: Early: Cloudiness of the cornea from the first post-op day. It is usually caused by defective donor endothelium or trauma during surgery. Late: Usually the result of immune graft rejection. 50 % occur in the first 6 months, and the majority occurs in the first year post-operatory.

It is equally important to know the history of allergies, systemic diseases and associations that can bring further complications in the recipient and ideally have the donor immunologic and systemic associations to verify their biocompatibility and immunological affinities between donor and receptor of the cornea. Another important issue is to verify early signs of rejection and microbiological differential diagnosis like infiltrates, edema, pain, to respond in time with the antibiotic, antifungal or antiviral indicated as appropriate in each case. Only in this way, it contributes to the success of a surgery that is vital to regain the vision and have no regrets later of rejection and putting at risk the integrity of visual health. Also, join efforts between expert around the world may compromise efforts against the rejection and the injury to prevent any complications and also to find new treatment options for actualize protocols, find new options and improve new technologies applied for medicine, engineering and new applications sciences for better quality life of patients.

6. Acknowledgment

To my friends: Doctor Emilio Méndez MD., Ophthalmologist, cornea specialist at Colombia, and Dr. Juliana Tirado MD., Ophthalmologist for their dedication to save corneas and contribute to research on ocular infections in our Country and to my co-workers of Research Group "Salud Visual" at Fundación Universitaria del Area Andina Pereira and our Institutional Research Center.

7. References

Barraquer, R.I., Alvarez, J.P, Fischer A. Martinez G., Prevención y tratamiento del asitigmatismo en queratoplastia penetrante. Annals d'oftalmologia 2002;10(2):69-80.

Buehler P O, Schein O D, Stamler J F, Verdier D D, Katz J. (1992). The increased risk of ulcerative keratitis among disposable soft contact lens users. *Arch Ophthalmol*; 110: 1555-8.
Butler KH, T. Dua, H. Edwards, R. James S. Lowe. (2001). In vitro model of crystalline infectious keratopaty : architecture of tissue determins the microbial propagation. *Investigative Ophthalmology & visual science*.2001. vol. 42 no. 6 1243-1.246.
Carringhton, LM, Albon J., Anderson I, Kamma C. Boulton M. (2006). Invest Ophthalmology Vis. Sci. May :47 (5) :1886-94.
Chalupa E, Swarbrick H, Holden B, Sjöstrand J. (1987). Severe corneal infections associated with contact lens wear. *Ophthalmology*; 94: 17-22.
Confino J, Brown SI. (1985). Bacterial endophthalmitis associated with exposed monofilament sutures following corneal transplantation. Am J Ophthalmol 99:111—3.
Cunnusamy, K. Chen PW, Niederkorn JY. (2010) Paradigm shifts in the role of CD+ T cells in keratoplasty. Discovery medicine. Nov;10 (54):452-61
Dana MR, Goren MB, Gomes JA, et al. (1995). Suture erosion after penetrating keratoplasty. *Cornea* 14:243—8.
Delgado, E., Durán, P., Neira O. y Veloza, G. (2008). Queratitis por Pseudomonas aeruginosa asociada al uso de lentes de contacto de hidrogel de silicona de última generación: Reporte de un caso. *Revista Chilena de Infectología*. 2008; 25 (4): 295-300.
Driebe WT, Stern GA. (1983). Microbial keratitis following corneal transplantation. *Cornea* 2:41.
Fong LP, Ormerod LD, Kenyon KR, et al.(1988). Microbial keratitis complicating penetrating keratoplasty. *Ophthalmology* 95:1269--75.
Fukuda, K., Yamada N., Fujitsu Y., Kumagai N. Nishida T.(2002). Inhibition of eatoxin expression in human corneal fibroblasts by IFN-gamma. International archives of allergies and immunology.
García Serrano, JL, Domínguez, Y, Serrano Laborda, D. (2004). Recurrencia de endoftalmitis bacteriana después de la queratoplastia penetrante. *Arch Soc Esp Oftalmol.*, vol.79, n.2, pp 89-92.
Gleich GJ, Adolphosn CR, Leiferman KM. The biology of the eosinophilic leukocite. Annu Rev Med 44 :85 - 101, 1993.
Hill R. (1976). The corneas need to breathe. *Int Contact Lens Clin*; 3: 60-1.
Holden B A, Sweeney D F, Sankaridurg P R, Camt N, Edwards K, Stretton S, et al. (2003). Microbial keratitis and vision loss with contact lenses. *Eye Contact Lens*; 29S: S131-4. discussion S143-4, S192-4.
Kumagai N, Fukuda K, Nishida T. (2005). Enhancement of conjunctival inflammation by corneal epithelial ablation in experimental allergic conjunctivitis. Presented in the Annual meeting 77ª of ARVO in Fort Lauderdale, Florida, May 1 - 5.
Kwong M, Evans D, Minjian N I, Cowell B, Fleiszig S. Human tear fluid protects against Pseudomonas aeruginosa keratitis in a murine experimental model.(2007). *Infect Immun* ; 75: 2325-32.
Maier, P. MD; F. Birnbaum, MD; Böhringer, D. MD; Reinhard, MD. (2010). Toxic Anterior Segment Syndrome Following Penetrating Keratoplasty. *Archieves of ophthalmology*. November 2.
Marquart M E, Caballero A R, Chomnawang M T, Brett A, Twining S S, O'Callaghan R J. (2005). Identification of a novel secreted protease from *Pseudomonas aeruginosa* that causes corneal erosions. *Invest Ophthalmol Vis Sci*; 46: 3761-8
McCulley JP, Alizadeh H, Niederkorn JY. (2000). The diagnosis and management of Acanthamoeba keratitis. *CLAO J* ;26:47-51.

Mertz G. (1980). Overnight swelling of the living human cornea. *J Am Optom Assoc*; 51: 211-4.

Miller M J, Ahearn D G. (1987). Adherence of Pseudomonas aeruginosa to hydrophilic contact lenses and other substrata. *J Clin Microbiol*; 25:1392-7.

Muzaliha Mohd Nor, Adil Hussein, Ibrahim Mohtar, Shatriah Ismail.(2010). Candida glabrata endophthalmitis following penetrating keratoplasty in a patient with negative donor rim culture. Department of Ophthalmology, School of Medical Sciences, Universiti Sains. Malaysia.

Nash, R. MD; Lindquist, Tomas, MD, PhD; Kalina, R. MD. (1991).An Evaluation of Saline Irrigation and Comparison of Povidone-Iodine and Antibiotic in the Surface Decontamination of Donor Eyes *Arco Ophthalmol.* ; 109 (6) :869-872.

Niederkorn JY, Alizadeh H, Leher HF, McCulley JP.(1999). The immunobiology of Acanthameoba keratitis. *Semin Immunopathol* ;21:147-60.

Poggio E C, Glynn R J, Schein O D, Seddon J M, Shannon M J, Scardino V A, et al. (1989).The incidence of ulcerative keratitis among users of daily-wear and extended - wear soft contact lenses. *N Engl J Med*; 321: 779-83.

Prakash G, Sharma N, Goel M, Titiyal JS, Vajpayee RB. (2008). Evaluation of Intrastromal Injection of Voriconazole as a Therapeutic Adjunctive for the Management of Deep Recalcitrant Fungal Keratitis. *Am J Ophthalmol*. Apr 23

Rasik B. Vajpayee, MS, FRCSEd, Namrata Sharma, MD, Rajesh Sinha, MD, FRCS, Tushar Agarwal, MD, and Arun Singhvi, MD. (2007). Infectious Keratitis Following Keratoplasty. *Survey of ophthalmology*. Volume 52 Number 1 January February.

Saxena, S, Kishore P, Pandey S, Khattri M, Kumar D. Topical bevacizumab for corneal noevascularization after penetrating keratoplasty. (2009). Eur. J. Ophthalmology. Sep Oct (5) :870-2

Shi, W., Wang T., Xie L. Li S, Gao H, Liu J, Li H. (2010) Risk factors, clinical features, and outcomes of recurrent fungal keratitis after corneal transplantation. State Key Laboratory Cultivation Base, Shandong Provincial Key Laboratory of Ophthalmology, Shandong Eye Institute, Qingdao, China. Epub Jan 15.

Sonavane A, MS, Sharma S., Gangopadhayay, N., Bansal A. (2003). Clinico-microbiologica correlation of suture-related graft infection following penetrating keratoplasty. *American Journal of Ophthalmology*. January.

Varga JH, Wolf TC, Jensen HG, Pamley VC, Rowsey JJ. (1993). Combined treatment of Acanthamoeba keratitis with propamidine, neomycin, and polyhexamethylene biguanide. *Am J Ophthalmol* ;115:466-70.

Wakimasu K, Sotozono C, Shimizu Y, Inatomi T, Sano Y, Nishida K, Yokoi N, Kinoshita S. (2004) A retrospective analysis of infection after corneal transplantation. Department of Ophthalmology, Kyoto Prefectural University Graduate School of Medicine, Japan. Nippon Ganka Gakkai Zasshi. Jun;108(6):354-8.

Xie L, Dong X, Shi W. (2001). Treatment of fungal keratitis by penetrating keratoplasty. Ophthalmol. Sep:85 (9):1070 – 4

You, Sonia H, Hurmeriv V. (2011). Femtosecond Lases-Assisted Keratoplasty. American Journal Of Ophthalmology. Vol 151, Issue 2

Zhu H, Thuruthyil S, Wilcox M D. (2002). Determination of quorum-sensing signal molecules and virulence factors of Pseudomonas aeruginosa isolates from contact lens-induced microbial keratitis. *J Med Microbiol*; 51: 1063-70.

8

Diagnosis and Treatment of a Rare Complication After Penetrating Keratoplasty: Retained Descemet's Membrane

Roberto Ceccuzzi, Gabriella Ricciardelli, Annita Fiorentino,
Meri Tasellari, Giovanni Furiosi and Paolo Emilio Bianchi
University of Pavia, Ophthalmic Department Foundation IRCCS San Matteo Pavia
Italy

1. Introduction

Retention of the host's Descemet's membrane is a complication which can occur during the course of a penetrating keratoplasty and which eventually leads to loss of graft clarity by clouding or by coming into contact with the graft endothelium. The retained Descemet's membrane can compromise endothelial tissue by contact injury or by limiting diffusion of aqueous humour nutrients.

In our study we discuss the pathogenesis, diagnosis and treatment of this complication. In addition we report some our cases treated with three different approaches.

2. Corneal transplant techniques

Corneal grafting techniques date back to the latter part of the 19th century and the earlier part of the 20th century as exemplified by pioneer ophthalmologists such as Reisinger, von Hippel and Elsching.

Penetrating Keratoplasty refers to the full thickness replacement of a diseased cornea with a healthy donor tissue. This technique may be used or to provide tectonic support in case of corneal thinning and perforation, either in case of keratoconus, bullous keratopathy, corneal dystrophies and degeneration, trauma or any other causes of corneal decompensation. Because of the "open sky" exposure of the intraocular contents during this kind of surgery, IOP control is an important step to avoid the risk of intraoperative expulsive choroidal haemorrhage. Using a calliper the horizontal and vertical diameters of the recipient's cornea are measured and the size of the graft is determined base on pathology and clinical judgement. Traditionally is used a size disparity in which the donor tissue is 0.25 mm larger than that of the recipient. The centre of the recipient cornea is marked so as the periphery with a radial keratotomy marker stained with ink. Then, while preparing the donor tissue punching the corneal button, the recipient cornea is cut by a trephine and the trephination is stopped as soon as aqueous egress shows the anterior chamber has been entered. Suction is released and the viscoelastic is then injected; the recipient button is excised using forceps and corneal scissors. Then the donor button is placed over the recipient bed and sutured in place with four cardinal sutures whose depth is typically 90% of the corneal thickness. After placement of the 12 o'clock suture, particular attention is paid to the 6 o'clock suture because these two sutures follow a vertical line and bisect the entire donor button such as the two at 3 and 9 o'clock. The rest of the sutures could be a combination of interrupted and running sutures.

But since the advent of penetrating keratoplasty surgeons have recognized the undesirable postoperative consequences of full-thickness corneal surgery such as high astigmatism, unpredictable refractive outcomes and prolonged visual rehabilitation. That's why ophthalmologists have conceptualized more selective transplanting techniques such as deep stromal and endothelial keratoplasty.

Lamellar keratoplasty involves placing a partial thickness donor corneal graft within a recipient corneal bed prepared by lamellar dissection of abnormal corneal tissue. It could be considered an alternative surgical option to penetrating keratoplasty in many specific cases such as all the ectactic corneal disorders that don't affect the endothelial cell layer. Lamellar keratoplasty offers several advantages over traditional PKP by avoiding complications associated with the "open sky" surgery and decreasing allograft rejection. The goal of this kind of surgery is a sufficient restoration of optical clarity of the central cornea; achievement of this objective is dependent upon a clean and complete posterior lamellar dissection of the host's corneal stroma from Descemet's membrane. An inadequate dissection could result in stromal and interface opacification and irregular astigmatism.

Descemet's stripping automatic endothelial keratoplasty (DSAEK) has become the preferred method of corneal transplantation for endothelial disease with improved safety, reduced astigmatism, and faster visual recovery. It is often performed with topical anaesthesia and monitored intravenous sedation. With the patient in a supine position, the horizontal corneal diameter of the recipient eye is measured with callipers to guide the selection of an appropriate donor tissue diameter. A 5 mm temporal clear corneal or sclera tunnel incision is made in the recipient eye. If the recipient epithelium is hazy or scarred it can be removed and this usually improves the view into the eye. Multiple ink points around the entire diameter of recipient cornea are used to lightly mark the surface of the recipient cornea to delineate the area for Descemet's membrane removal. The recipient endothelium, in fact, should only be stripped from the area that will be covered by the donor tissue because any stripped area not covered with donor tissue will become oedematous. To prevent this occurrence some surgeons score an area somewhat smaller than the planned donor diameter. Trypan blue could also be introduced in the anterior chamber to improve membrane visualization during the stripping. Descemet's membrane is then scored in a circular pattern along the perimeter of the area to be removed with a modified hook. During the scoring and stripping steps the anterior chamber can remain formed by continuous infusion of balanced salt solution or air (we prefer to avoid the use of viscoelastic because, if it will not be completely removed before inserting the donor button, it will impair donor adherence).

After the donor tissue is inserted the anterior chamber is inflated by injecting air or balanced salt solution which allows the posterior portion of the donor tissue to unfold. The anterior chamber is then completely filled with air to firmly press the donor tissue up against the recipient cornea.

3. Retention of Descemet's membrane

Retention of the host's Descemet's membrane is a complication which can occur during the course of a penetrating keratoplasty (but also DALK and DSAEK present retention of Descemet's complications) and which eventually leads to loss of graft clarity by clouding or by coming into contact with the graft endothelium. Penetrating keratoplasty is a common technique with good prognosis value and has been the first choice for corneal endothelial decompensation even if in the last years for this kind of diseases DSAEK is preferred in order to its minimal sequelae. DSAEK requires much less manipulation of the recipient cornea and anterior chamber, compared with the earlier PK and DALK procedure and this help to minimize intraoperative and postoperative complications. Moreover DSAEK technique does not induce significative alterations of corneal topography so that it could be considered an essentially refractive neutral transplant procedure.

Postoperative complications of penetrating keratoplasty include high or irregular astigmatism, prolonged wound healing, late wound dehiscence with trauma, suture-related infections, vascularisation, and graft rejection. The most postoperative complication with DSAEK, instead, is that sometimes the donor tissue detaches in the early postoperative period (from 1 day to 1 week after surgery) so that additional air must to be injected to again firmly press the donor tissue against the recipient cornea.

In addition, retention of the host's Descemet's membrane can be seen as a rare complication of these surgical techniques. The retained Descemet's membrane can compromise endothelial tissue by contact injury or by limiting diffusion of aqueous humour nutrients.

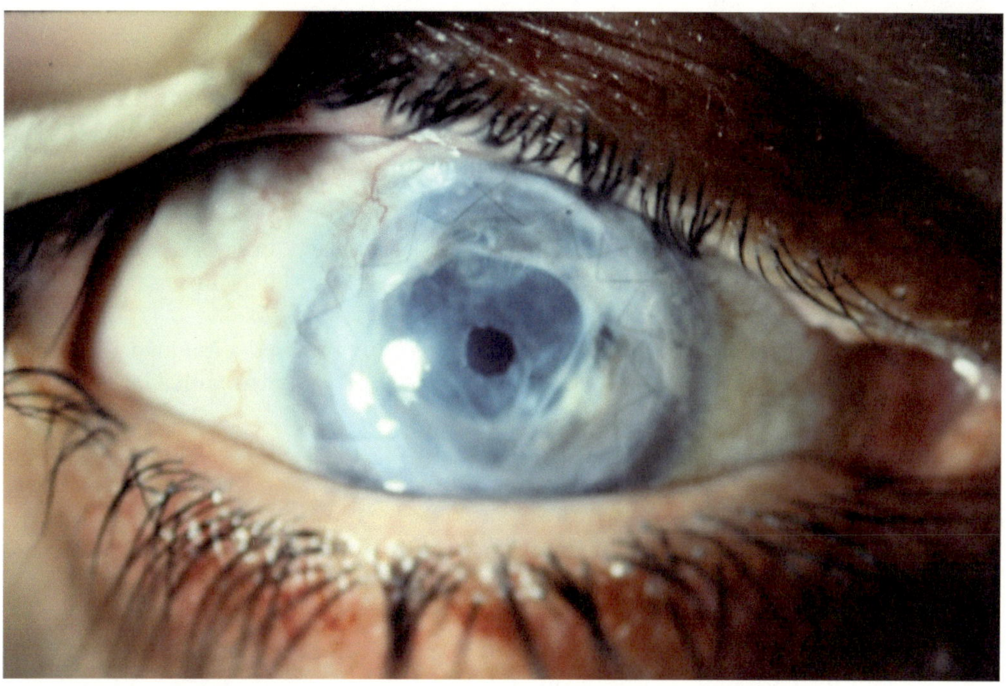

Fig. 1.a Retained Descemet's membrane after PK treated with YAG laser

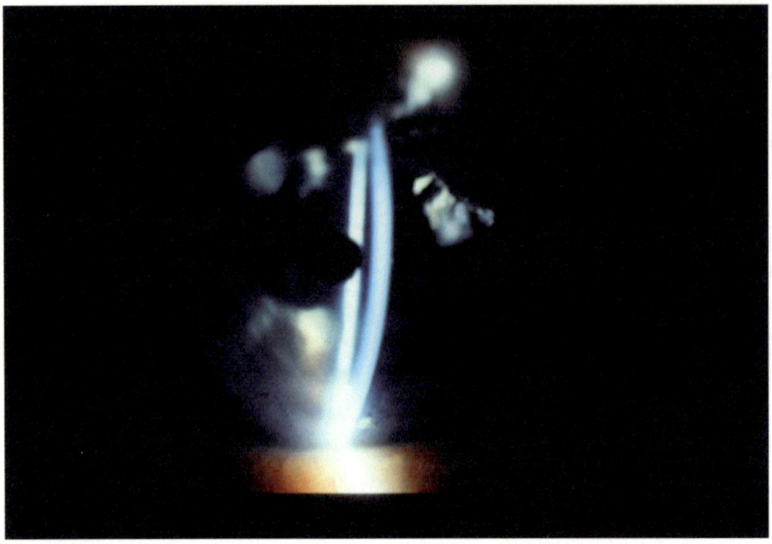

Fig. 1.b Retained Descemet's membrane after PK treated with YAG laser

This complication consists in the incomplete removal of the host cornea: after partial trephination we make an opening into the anterior chamber and introduce curved corneal scissors. Especially in an oedematous cornea it could occur that the lower blade is placed anterior to Descemet's membrane so that, when the button is lifted from the eye, a portion of Descemet's membrane leaves behind.

The result is a wavy, diaphanous membrane that creates a supernumerary anterior chamber behind the graft on the first postoperative control by slit lamp examination.

The following case histories from the Department of Ophthalmology of San Matteo General Hospital of Pavia, may help to illustrate the course and prognosis of this mishap.

4. Cases report

4.1 Case 1

A 62 year old white woman underwent penetrating keratoplasty in her right eye on April 23, 2002. Because of the appearance of deep new vessels, especially in nasal and upper corneal sectors, she underwent a retransplantation on February 26, 2003.

On the first post-operative control, slit lamp biomicroscopy revealed a retained Descemet's membrane and a supernumerary anterior chamber. The graft was clear with a best corrected visual acuity of 1/10 with +2 D sphere.

The patient opted for Laser treatment (March 2003) to improve visual function so that it was created a central circular opening in the retrograft membrane at optical zone level just one month after PK.

The laser was setted to 0.9 mJ with posterior focus shift and increased up to 1.7 mJ when a central tear appeared in the membrane; subsequently enlarged focusing the beam near to the first tear to create a central circular 2.5 mm opening.

There were no complication resulting from the Yag Laser treatment and the donor cornea remained thin and clear with a visual acuity two years after PK improved to 6/10 with +2 D sphere.

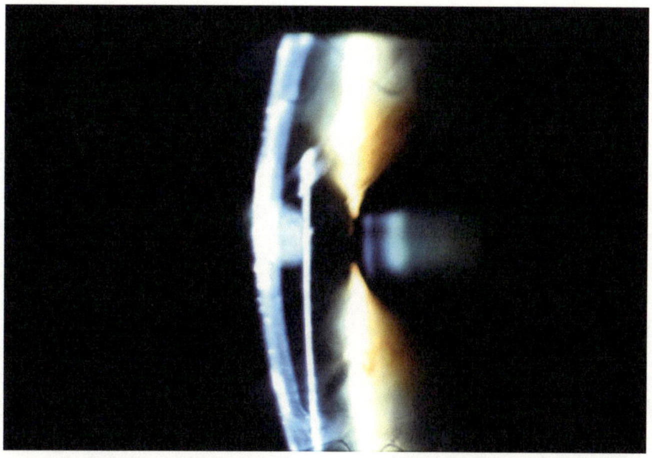

Fig. 2. Partial double anterior chamber in retained Descemet's membrane

4.2 Case 2

A 54 year old white woman was referred to our department on December 2002. The patient was diagnosed as having glaucoma in 1990 and since than on she was treated with Timololo.
In 1998 a cataract extraction was performed in patient's right eye and on December 03, 2002 she underwent a penetrating keratoplasty in RE for endothelial decompensation. After surgery the patient reported excellent visual function lasting for some time but on July 2003 she had experienced decreased visual acuity and marked diffuse corneal oedema, later on which it was performed a retransplantation.
On the first post-operative control the slit lamp biomicroscopy revealed a Descemet's retention with a supernumerary anterior chamber so that the patient underwent descemetorhexis to leave the pupillary field one month later. Nine months after the treatment the patient had a best-corrected visual acuity of 5/10 and the graft was clear. Unfortunately the patient did not complete the follow-up in our department.

4.3 Case 3

An 81 year old man with a history of cataract extraction in both eyes, glaucoma and penetrating keratoplasty in right eye in 2000, was referred to the Department of Ophthalmology of San Matteo General Hospital with ocular pain and marked reduction of visual acuity. In spite of risks connected with his glaucomatous history, the patient opted for new surgical treatment and on October 2003 he underwent a new penetrating keratoplasty.
On the first post-operative control was referred Descemet's retention from removed graft. On September 2004 the graft appeared oedematous and with a lot of new vessels all around the limbus. Because of this on November 23, 2004 was performed a new penetrating keratoplasty in right eye. On the last control (September 2010) the patient's visual acuity in his right eye was limited to hand motions.

5. Discussion

These cases document the occurrence of a retained Descemet's membrane following penetrating keratoplasty especially in case of severe oedema and thickening of the recipient cornea, which facilitates the separation of Descemet's membrane and, in turn, incomplete trephination when the recipient cornea is cut. Alternatively, it can be caused by improper instillation of a viscoelastic agent, which can dissect an artificial corneal plane and contribute to inadvertent retention of posterior corneal lamellae.

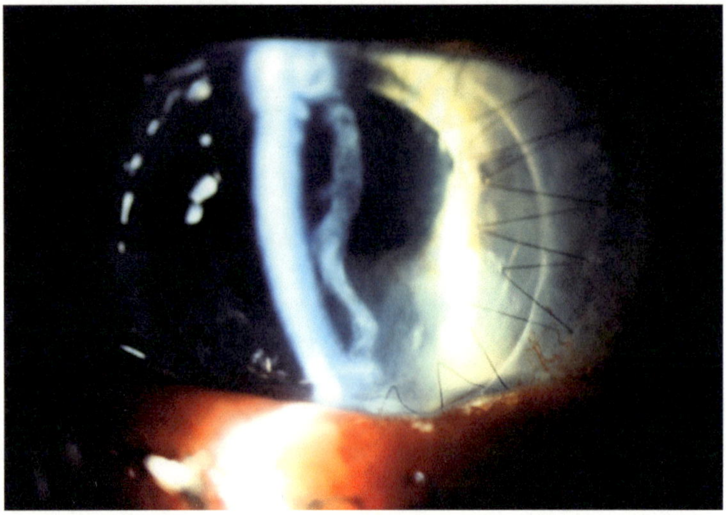

Fig. 3. Double anterior chamber in retained Descemet's membrane

The principal mechanisms which lead to Descemet's membrane's retention are:

- inadvertent and incomplete trephination of oedematous corneas as in congenital hereditary endothelial dystrophy or bullous keratopathy that forces the surgeon to complete the cut with forceps acting on different levels;
- longstanding stromal oedema which cause loosening of the attachment of the DM, thereby predisposing to its separation from the overlying stroma
- marked hypotonia of ocular globe with decrease of backpressure during the cut
- scar's marked fibrosis in case of retransplantation
- stromal recipient imbibitions (not by chance in some techniques of DALK surgery the imbibitions is deliberately requested to make easier the identification of Descemet's membrane). It's important to underline that in case of corneal imbibitions Descemet's membrane becomes thickened due to endothelial decompensation and this fact leads to a further resistance to trephination.

The retained DM may be associated with progressive opacification of the graft that has been postulated to occur due to presence of a sliver of residual stroma with keratocytes from which the fibroblastic activity occurs. The differential time taken for the opacification of the retained DM is due to the thickness of the residual stroma retained along with the DM in these cases.

The best way to avoid this complication is to inspect the wound site carefully with the operating microscope at high magnification and pick up the iris with a fine-tipped forceps to detect a detached Descemet's membrane, especially in oedematous corneal host tissue.

Also, it is important to note that loss of aqueous humour during trephination indicates Descemet's membrane is perforated in 1 or more places, even if this doesn't strictly mean that Descemet's membrane has been completely cut.

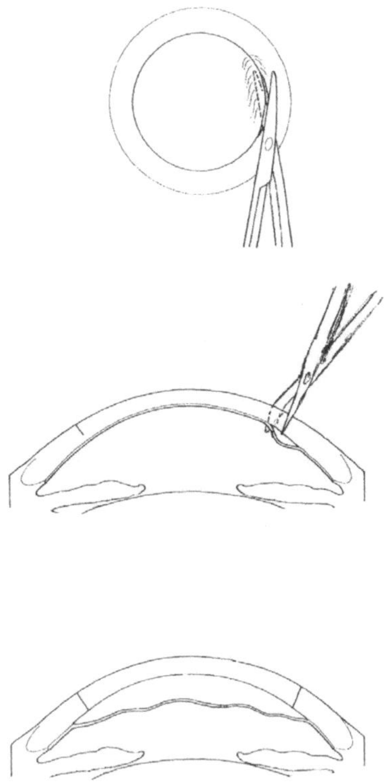

Fig. 4. Scissors incomplete insertion results in retained Descemet's membrane

A possible solution to this problem is the use of dye, such as trypan blue or indocyanine green, to highlight the Descemet's membrane. The use of indocyanine green staining of the Descemet's membrane to make DLEK surgery easier has previously been described. Although it bears further study to determine its value, the use of dye after Descemet's stripping in DSEK may improve visualization of this transparent membrane and alleviate the inadvertent retention of the delaminated fetal Descemet's membrane on the recipient bed.

About DALK surgery it's possible to have retained Descemet's in management of a complication such as macroperforation and subsequently surgical switch to PKP in critical condition: shallow anterior chamber, poor surgical field vision for stromal air or fluid imbibition, dishomogeneous thickness due to the pathology (often keratoconus).

Even during DSAEK Descemet's retention could be a complication which affects the outcome of corneal surgery. Crucial is in this case the presence of folded peripheral spurs that prevent the attachment of donor button being responsible of graft failure. In this case AS-OCT is a useful instrument for the early recognition of retained Descemet's membrane. Retained Descemet's membrane after keratoplasty can be difficult to diagnose in the early postoperative course and AS-OCT may be a useful adjunctive diagnostic tool to aid in the recognition and management of such a complication, especially for patients with either corneal opacity or oedema or after corneal surgeries.

To determine whether the entire desired surgical area of the Descemet's membrane has been removed in DSEK surgery, practitioners routinely examine the stripped Descemet's membrane during surgery with placement of the tissue onto the anterior corneal surface.

Doing so allows the surgeon to visually inspect the tissue for missing fragments, which could be removed from the anterior chamber. Despite this precaution, it would be difficult, if not impossible, for the surgeon to discern whether a small lamellar remnant was retained on the recipient's posterior cornea.

Retention of the host's Descemet's membrane is a complication which can occur during the course of a penetrating keratoplasty and which eventually leads to loss of graft clarity by clouding or by coming into contact with the graft endothelium. The retained Descemet's membrane can compromise endothelial tissue by contact injury or by limiting diffusion of aqueous humour nutrients. That's why the use of YAG laser could allow not only the optic zone relief but also the diffusion of aqueous humour nutrients, avoiding complications related to retransplantation. Moreover this "non open sky" technique grants us smaller risk of postoperative complications but avoids only a little central hole which results inadequate in case of big descemetical residue. We have also to notice that Yag laser could induce a further Descemet's - endothelial failure thanks to its thermic effect.

6. References

Archila E.A., Ramirez Cabrera M.F. Alviar A.M., Double Descemt's Membrane in Penetrating Keratoplasty *J Refract and Corneal Surg. 9 65-66, 1993*

Banik R, Novick LH, Smith RE, & Chuck RS. Retrocorneal Membrane With Descemet's Detachment *Cornea* 20(7): 763–764, 2001

Bui K.M., Tu E.Y. *A R*igid Band of Retained Descemet's Membrane as a Mechanical Cause of Graft Non-attachment in Repeat DSAEK. ARVO 2011 Abstract - May 1-5 2011

Chen YP, Lai PCC, Chen PYF, Lin KK, & Hsiao CH. Retained Descemet's membrane after penetrating keratoplasty *J Cataract Refract* Surg 2003; 29:1842–1844

Cohen AV, Goins KM, Sutphin JE, Wandling GR, & Wagoner MD. Penetrating keratoplasty versus deep anterior lamellar keratoplasty for the treatment of keratoconus. *Int Ophthalmol* (2010) 30:675–681

Ichihashi Y., Nejima R., Matsumoto Y., Kawakita T., Miyata K., Tsubota K., Shimmura S. Results of Non-Descemet's Stripping And Automated Endothelial Keratoplasty (nDSAEK) ARVO 2011 Abstract - May 1-5 2011

Ide T., Yoo S.H., Kymionis G.D., Shah P. A., & O'Brien T. P.. Double Descemet's Membranes After Penetrating Keratoplasty With Anterior Segment Optical Coherence Tomography *Ophthalmic surgery laser and imaging* 2008; 39, 05: 422-425

Mittal V, Mittal R, & Sangwan VS. Successful Descemet's stripping endothelial keratoplasty in congenital hereditary endothelial dystrophy *Cornea* 2011 Mar;30(3):354-356

Mondloch M. C., Giegengack M., Terry M. A. & Wilson D. J. Histologic Evidence of Retained Fetal Layer of the Descemet's Membrane After Presumed Total Removal for Endothelial Keratoplasty A Possible Cause for Graft Failure *Cornea* 2007; 26, 10: 1263-1266

Romaniv N., Price M.O., Price F. W., & Nick Mamalis. Donor Descemet's Membrane Detachment After Endothelial Keratoplasty *Cornea* 2006; 25, 8: 943-947

Sbarbaro JA, Eagle RC, Thumma P, & Raber IM. Histopathology of Posterior Lamellar Endothelial Keratoplasty Graft Failure *Cornea* 2008;27:900–904

9

Topical Bevacizumab Therapy in Graft Rejection After Penetrating Keratoplasty

Sandeep Saxena and Neha Sinha
Department of Ophthalmology, C.S.M. Medical University (Erstwhile King George's Medical University) Lucknow, India

1. Introduction

Neovascularization is defined as formation of new vessels from vascular endothelial cells derived from existing blood vessels. These new immature vessels are friable. They have increased permeability, lack structural integrity, and can result in lipid deposition and corneal opacities. Ultrastructurally, corneal neovascularization is characterized by vessels encroaching through separated stromal lamellae. Corneal vascularization following penetrating keratoplasty may result in graft rejection.

2. Pathophysiology

Angiogenesis is a complex processs. First, inflammatory mediators trigger vasodilation and increase vascular permeability of limbal and conjunctival vasculature. Vascular endothelial growth factor (VEGF) is one of the most important regulators of corneal angiogenesis. It is produced primarily by macrophages, T cells, and smooth muscle cells in ocular surface.

A second important regulator of corneal neovascularization is basic fibroblast growth factor (bFGF) and the third important signal is platelet aggregation factor (PAF). Others include insulin like growth factor, integrins, transforming growth factor, tumor necrosis factor and matrix metalloproteinase.

Corneal neovascularization can be prevented by various anti angiogenic factors that have been identified in the cornea. Angiostatin, a proteolytic fragment of plasminogen prevents neovascularization and also induces regression of existing vessels. This has been identified in chronic contact lens user where it suppresses the angiogenic stimuli of hypoxia. Second antiangiogenic factor is endostatin which is a proteolytic fragment of collagen XVIII inhibits bFGF and VEGF stimulated corneal neovascularization. Third naturally occurring antiangiogenic factor is pigment epithelium derived growth factor (PEDF) which is a serine protease inhibitor and inhibits bFGF stimulated corneal neovascularization.

Corneal neovascularization most frequently results from corneal oxygen deprivation, or hypoxia. In response to this hypoxia, the body attempts to provide necessary nutrients and oxygen to the deprived corneal tissues by the creation of new blood vessels. During the early stages, this abnormal growth of blood vessels may produce no signs at all, or it may cause a variety of symptoms, including eye pain and excessive tearing, light sensitivity, redness, intolerance to contact lenses, and decreased vision.

Role of Corneal Neovascularization in Corneal Graft Rejection

Corneal neovascularization remains a significant risk factor for corneal graft rejection and subsequent graft failure after penetrating keratoplasty. The collaborative corneal transplantation study[1] identified, in addition to several other factors, the extent of stromal vessels (quadrants) as a serious risk factor for corneal graft failure. During corneal neovascularization, an upregulation of angiogenic factors is seen in association with down regulation of antiangiogenic molecules. Studies in human and rat models have found vascular endothelial growth factor (VEGF) to be up regulated in inflamed and vascularized cornea .[2] In a mouse model, it was observed that corneal avascularity during development is redundantly regulated. Lack of the antiangiogenic factors thrombospondin (TSP)-1 and/or -2 resulted in no spontaneous corneal angiogenesis. By contrast, TSP-1, more than TSP-2, helped to suppress inflammation-induced corneal angiogenesis postnatally, implying that angiogenic privilege in the cornea is actively maintained .[3] Bachmann et al[4] in a mouse model found that neutralization of VEGF-A after high-risk corneal transplantation effectively inhibited postoperative hemangiogenesis, lymphangiogenesis, and recruitment of antigen-presenting cells, thereby improving corneal graft survival.

Vascular endothelial growth factor promotes several steps of angiogenesis, including proteolytic activities, endothelial cell proliferation, migration, and capillary tube formation . [5] Topical or systemic application of bevacizumab inhibited both inflammation-induced angiogenesis and lymphangiogenesis in the cornea. This finding suggestes an important role of VEGF-A in corneal lymphangiogenesis and bevacizumab may be useful in preventing immune rejections after penetrating keratoplasty.

3. Types of corneal vascularization

Superficial: In superificial corneal vascularization, vessels arrange in arborizing pattern in subepithelial layer and can be traced with conjunctival vessels. This type of vascularization may be observed in trachoma, and phlyctenular conjunctivitis.

Deep: In deep corneal vascularization, vessels are derived from anterior ciliary artery and lie in corneal stroma. Vessels are usually straight and not anastomosing. This type of vascularization may be observed in graft rejection, interstitial keratitis, deep corneal ulcer, and chemical burn.

Pannus: In pannus, extensive superficial vascularization occurs with cellular infiltration. It is of two types:

- Progressive: Infiltration is ahead of vascularization
- Regressive: Infiltration is behind the vascular leash.

4. Associated symptoms

Symptoms of corneal neovascularization often include the following:

- Eye pain
- Redness
- Tearing and photophobia

- Contact lens intolerance
- Decreased vision

4.1 Advantages of neovascularization
- Transport humoral and cellular elements of immunological defence and raw material
- Repair and regeneration
- Carry antibiotic and drugs to site of infection
- Eliminates toxic substances

4.2 Disadvantages of neovascularization
- Interfere with corneal transparency
- Graft rejection and failure in keratoplasty
- Sensitization to other antigen

4.3 Complications
- Corneal edema
- Corneal opacity
- Graft rejection in keratoplasty
- Lipid keratopathy
- Intrastromal/subepithelial bleeding
- It can also lead to blindness

5. Management

Corneal neovascularization is one of the main risk factor for immune rejection after corneal transplantation. Healthy cornea is devoid of blood vessels and is said to be immune privileged. When corneal grafts are placed into an avascular recipient corneal bed (*low risk keratoplasty*) the two year survival rate approaches 90% under cover of steroids.

The survival rates of corneal grafts placed over vascularized recipient beds (*high risk keratoplasty*) decrease significantly. Even in low risk setting, mild angiogenesis develops after keratoplasty and increase risk of immune graft rejection. For this reason aggressive treatment of neovascularization may be necessary prior to corneal transplant surgery to ensure lower risk of graft rejection.

Various antiangiogenic agents may be used in management of post keratoplasty graft rejection:

- Angiostatic steroids
- Vascular endothelial growth factor inhibitor
- Protein kinase c inhibitor
- MMP inhibitor
- COX-2 inhibitor
- Antioxidants
- Dietary derived inhibitor

Corticosteroids and systemic immunosuppression remain an important aspect in prevention of post keratoplasty graft rejection. Corticosteroids inhibit macrophages that release growth

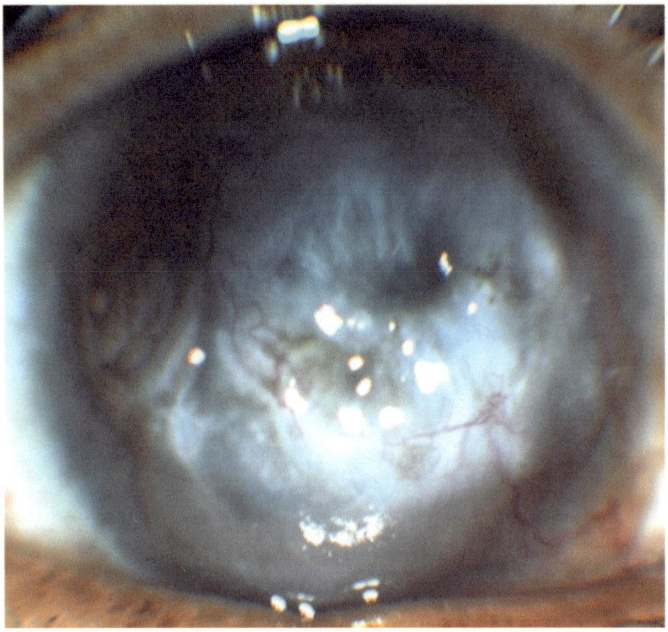

A

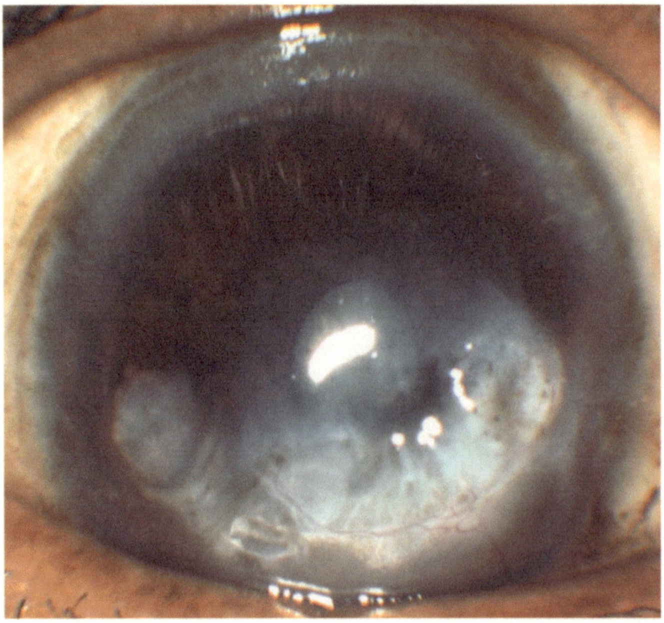

B

Fig. 1. Effect of topical bevacizumab in a case of corneal neovascularization. A. Pre-treatment: Corneal vascularization and stromal haze is visible. B. Post-treatment: Marked regression in corneal vascularization and stromal haze has resulted.

factor. They also prevent intercellular adhesion leading to leukocyte adhesion and migration. They can slow the progression of neovascularization, but cannot stabilize or reverse the process.

Vascular endothelial growth factor inhibitors are emerging as the new pharmacological therapy in the management of post keratoplasty graft rejection. Anti-VEGF agent has been found to be effective in reducing corneal vascularization (Fig. 1). Currently available anti-VEGF agents include:

- **Bevacizumab (Avastin)** Bevacizumab is a humanized monoclonal antibody that inhibits all active isoforms of VEGF and is approved by USFDA since February 2004 for treatment of metastatic colorectal cancer.
- **Ranibizumab (Lucentis)** Ranibizumab is also a humanized monoclonal antibody fragment highly related to bevacizumab structurally.
- **Pegaptanib (Macugen)** Pegaptanib is a synthetic oligonucleotide that binds the pathologic isoform of VEGF, which is VEGF 165 and this binding, happens extracellular.

5.1 Role of bevacizumab in the treatment of corneal vascularization

Efficacy of bevacizumab therapy has been highlighted in several studies. Manzano et al [6] in an experimental study on rats showed that a concentration of 4 mg/mL bevacizumab limits corneal neovascularization. Dastjerdi et al[7] in their study used 1% bevacizumab for 3 weeks in 10 eyes of 10 patients and followed them up to 24 weeks. They found that short-term topical bevacizumab therapy reduced the severity of corneal neovascularization without local or systemic adverse effects. Chen et al[8] used subconjunctival injection of bevacizumab in doses 0.25-2.5 mg twice per week for 2 to 8 weeks in rabbits and concluded that it is effective in preventing corneal neovascularization in acute phase of various kinds of corneal inflammation. Carrasco [9] reported the use of bevacizumab in an 81-year old woman with corneal neovascularization secondary to herpetic stromal keratitis. Treatment with subconjunctival bevacizumab showed regression of corneal neovascularization. Bock et al[10] in their study used topical bevacizumab (5x/day; 5 mg/ml) for 15 days in corneal neovascularization of various cause and concluded that it inhibits corneal neovascularization without obvious corneal epithelial side effects.

5.2 Role of bevacizumab in the treatment of corneal vascularization after keratoplasty

Efficacy of bevacizumab therapy has been highlighted in several studies. Schollmayer et al[11] performed a retrospective case series study of nine eyes of nine patients with corneal transplant and neovascularization. Five eyes were administered topical bevacizumab 5 mg/ml 4 times daily for a month. Three eyes were administered bevacizumab subconjunctivally 2.5 mg/0.1 ml and one eye was administered bevacizumab both topically as well via subconjunctival route. After a follow up of 6 months, it was concluded that topical and subconjunctival bevacizumab is effective in regressing neovascularization in keratoplasty patients.

Saxena et al[12] used topical bevacizumab (4 mg/4 ml) in dose of one drop twice daily for 15 days in a patient of corneal graft rejection and did a follow up after 1 month, 6 month and 9 months. After 1 month, his BCVA improved to 20/120 from finger counting 1meter. Corneal vascularization and stromal haze regressed. After 6 months, his BCVA improved to 20/60

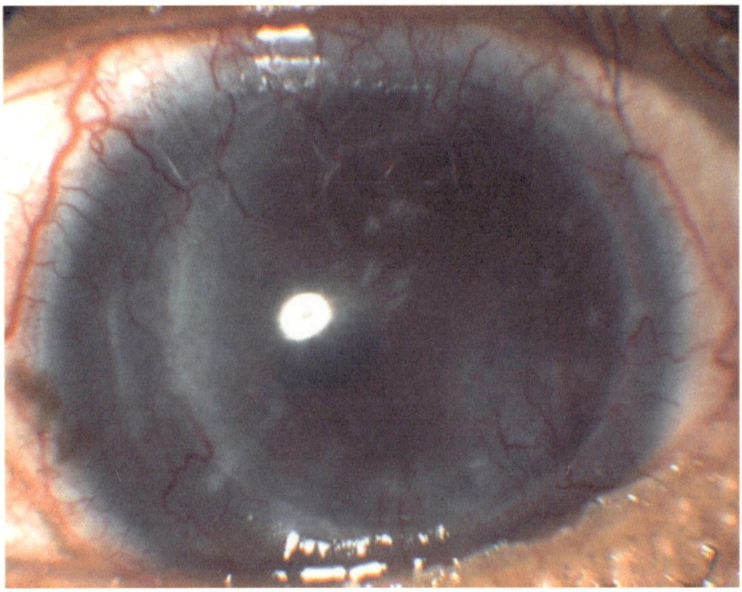

A

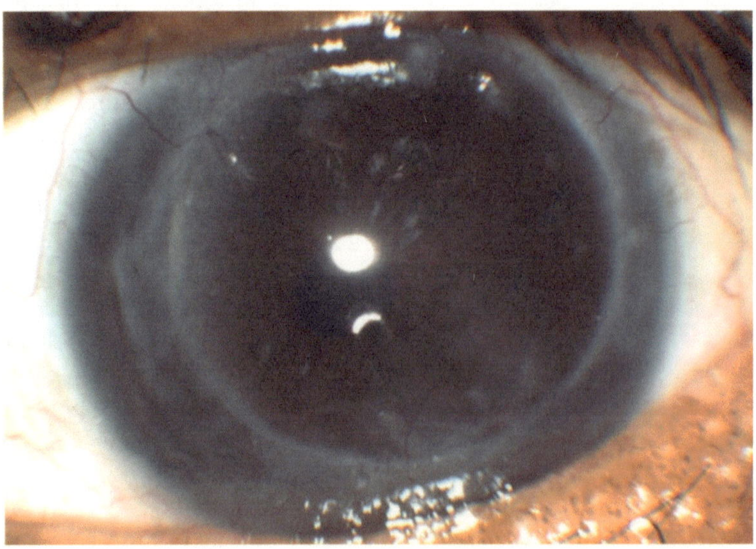

B

Fig. 2. Effect of topical bevacizumab on corneal neovasculariszation in a post-keratoplasty patient. A. Pre-treatment: Severe corneal vascularization and stromal haze is present. B. Post-treatment: Marked regression of corneal vascularization and reduction of stromal haze is observed

with further regression in corneal vascularization and stromal haze resulted. At 9-month follow-up, he maintained BCVA of 20/60. Thus they concluded that short-term topical bevacizumab therapy may potentially offer a safer and more effective alternative in treating graft rejection after penetrating keratoplasty (Fig. 2).
Despite effective results, corneal thinning and epithelial defect following topical bevacizumab instillation has also been reported.[13]

6. Conclusion

Although limited number of studies are available in literature, growing evidence suggests that bevacizumab offers a safe and effective mode of treatment for graft rejection following penetrating keratoplasty.

7. References

[1] Maguire MG, Stark WJ, Gottsch JD, et al. Risk factors for corneal graft failure and rejection in collaborative corneal transplantation studies: Collaborative Corneal Transplantation Studies Research Group. Ophthalmology. 1994; 101: 1536-1547.

[2] Philipp W, Speicher L, Humpel C. Expression of vascular endothelial growth factor and its receptors in inflamed and vascularised human corneas. Invest Ophthalmol Vis Sci. 2000;41: 2514-2522.

[3] Cursiefen C, Masli S, Fong T, et al. Roles of thrombospondin- 1 and -2 in regulating corneal and iris angiogenesis. Invest Ophthalmol Vis Sci. 2004; 45: 1117-1124.

[4] Bachmann BO, Bock F, Wiegand SJ, et al. Promotion of graft survival by vascular endothelial growth factor-A neutralization after high-risk corneal transplantation. Arch Ophthalmol. 2008; 126: 71-77.

[5] Erdurmus M, Totan Y. Subconjunctival bevacizumab for corneal neovascularisation. Graefes Arch Clin Exp Ophthalmol 2007; 245: 1577-1579.

[6] Manzano RPA, Peyman GA, Khan P, Petros E, Kivilcim CM, Ren M, et al. Br J Ophthalmol. 2007;91:804-807.

[7] Dastjerdi MH, Al-Arfaj KM, Nallasamy N, Hamrah P, Jurkunas UV, Pineda R 2nd, et al. Arch Ophthalmol. 2009;127:381-389.

[8] Wei-Li Chen W , Chung-Tien Lin, Nien-Ting Lin, et al. Bevacizumab on corneal neovascularisation in different rabbit models of corneal angiogenesis. Invest Ophthalmol Vis Sci 2010 51:6277-6285.

[9] Carrasco MA. Subconjunctival bevacizumab for corneal neovascularization in herpetic stromal keratitis Cornea. 2008;27: 743-745.

[10] Bock F, König Y, Kruse F, Baier M, Cursiefen C. Bevacizumab eyedrops inhibit corneal neovascularization. Graefe's Arch Clin Exp Ophthalmol. 2008; 246: 281-284.

[11] Schollmayer P, Stunf S, Lavric A. Pfeifer V. Topical and subconjunctival bevacizumab in corneal neovascularization in keratoplasty patients. Acta Ophthalmologica, 2008;86: 0. doi: 10.1111/j.1755-3768.2008.570.x

[12] Saxena S, Kishore P, Pandey S, Khattri M, Kumar D. Topical bevacizumab for corneal neovascularization after penetrating keratoplasty.Eur J Ophthalmol. 2009;19:870-872.

[13] Kim SW, Ha BJ, Kim EK, Tchah H, Kim TI. The effect of topical bevacizumab on corneal neovascularisation. Ophthalmology. 2008;115:E33-8.